YOUR LIFE TO ENJOY

Peter J. Steincrohn, M.D.

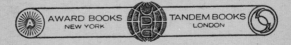

AWARD BOOKS
NEW YORK

TANDEM BOOKS
LONDON

FIRST AWARD PRINTING 1970

DEDICATION

To my wife Patti and my daughter Barbara

Copyright © MCMLXIII by Peter J. Steincrohn, M.D.

Published by arrangement with Prentice-Hall, Inc.

All rights reserved

Library of Congress Catalog Number: 63-12273

AWARD BOOKS are published by
Universal-Award House, Inc., a subsidiary of
Universal Publishing and Distributing Corporation,
235 East Forty-fifth Street, New York, N.Y. 10017

TANDEM BOOKS are published by
Universal-Tandem Publishing Company Limited
14 Gloucester Road, London SW7, England

Manufactured in the United States of America

TRUE OR FALSE?

- There is no more harm in tobacco than in a cup of tea
- Liquor is good for you
- It's good to be a hypochondriac
- Drugs are less harmful than anxiety
- You can rest in a hammock and still remain fit
- The role of cholesterol in heart and artery disease has not been established
- You may be killing your body with kindness

If you answered *false* to any of these, you may want to answer again—after you've read this book.

"Eat, drink and be healthy," is Dr. Steincrohn's advice "because there is no valid, sensible reason to live over-cautiously."

The only way to keep your health is to eat what you don't want, drink what you don't like, and do what you'd rather not.

MARK TWAIN

To keep well by too strict a regimen is a tedious disease in itself.

LA ROCHEFOUCAULD

Every man who knows how to read has it in his power to magnify himself, to multiply the ways in which he exists, to make his life full, significant, and interesting.

ALDOUS HUXLEY

Contents

Introduction

Forget the Ten

Health Commandments

Don't do this?

Don't do that?

Recently, a business man said, "Whenever I visit my doctor my conscience is heavy. I rarely leave his office feeling that I have been a cooperative patient. In fact, I have developed the 'bad boy complex.' It seems everything I do is wrong."

People are getting fed up and rebellious at having to listen to so many "don'ts." Soon patients will be like those negativistic unmanageable youngsters who rebel at anything and everything you tell them or ask them to do. They are becoming so tired of being admonished: "don't do this" and "better not do that"—their ears will soon be closed to any good suggestions whatever.

For example, here is a man who enjoys moderate smoking. We raise doubts and spectres of doom, telling him he will *surely* get cancer of the lung if he doesn't quit. *Surely?*

Here is another who has limited himself to an ounce or

11

two of liquor a day for over 30 years, yet has not succumbed to chronic alcoholism. However, his doctor says, "Better stop drinking. You don't want to get cirrhosis of the liver, do you?" *Surely?*

Likewise we are warned about the dangers of getting too fat, of not exercising enough, of taking too much cholesterol. Lately there even have been reports that eating smoked foods may predispose to cancer of the stomach. At least not *surely?*

Think how much we live in confusion, indecision and anxiety.

Consider the many thousands who are befuddled by the cholesterol problem. They feed themselves as if they were robots, not human beings.

Consider the reducing-diet fads which transform us into a nation of silly, starved sheep.

Consider your own guilt complex when you choose to relax in a hammock or chair rather than "be out exercising as you should."

Consider how moralizing interferes when you reach for a martini.

Consider the people who are "afraid" they are drinking too much tea or coffee.

Consider how anxiety disturbs the sublime pleasure of the after-dinner cigar; how statistics ruin the comfort of the cigarette smoker; how guilty the pipe smoker feels when he is told that his addiction is due to an infantile residuum to suck on something.

Recall your recent visits to your doctor and you will agree that lately we have gotten into the habit of telling you what **not** to do rather than what to **do.** We issue our sermons on health in the form of Commandments cast in negative form—because it is easier to tell people what not to do than what to do.

For example, here are **Ten Health Commandments** (among others) we doctors issue. Every day, in offices throughout the United States millions of patients hear these decrees:

1. THOU SHALT NOT TAKE CHOLESTEROL
2. THOU SHALT NOT BE LAZY
3. THOU SHALT NOT TAKE TOBACCO
4. THOU SHALT NOT TAKE ALCOHOL
5. THOU SHALT NOT EAT TOO MUCH
6. THOU SHALT NOT HAVE ANXIETY
7. THOU SHALT NOT BE UNDER TOO GREAT STRESS
8. THOU SHALT NOT BECOME A VICTIM OF YOUR EMOTIONS
9. THOU SHALT NOT HAVE TOO MANY DOCTORS
10. THOU SHALT NOT RETIRE FROM YOUR JOB TOO EARLY

Nevertheless, cheer up! In spite of all these and similar restrictions, you need not buckle under. Conformity is one of the major ills of our age. Do everything you can **not** to come down with this deadening sickness. Though all the others be sheep, see if you can be lion-hearted. Honest rebelliousness is refreshing in this time of fear, anxiety and half-living.

Remember that most people can eat all kinds of sweets yet do not get diabetes. Others eat many varieties of fats yet don't have high cholesterol levels. Others smoke and have no ill effects. Many can "eat nails" yet have no stomach trouble. Hundreds of thousands, under severe daily stresses, never get high blood pressure or ulcers or heart disease. The majority drink yet never become chronic alcoholics.

Nevertheless, many would be willing to forego creamed onions, fine steaks, rich desserts—if they were *certain* that having a normal cholesterol level in the blood would protect them from having a coronary attack or stroke.

You would go without smoking—at a great sacrifice to your personal comfort—if you could be *certain* that tobacco was the real cause of cancer of the lungs and deterioration of your arteries.

You would go without drinking if you were *certain* that becoming an abstainer would spare your liver and heart.

You would reduce—giving up your pizzas, favorite French pastries, among other snacks—if you were *certain* that obesity was endangering your life.

You would try to control your temper if you were *certain* that, by preventing emotional outbursts, you could prevent a vessel bursting in your brain or a clogged artery in your heart.

You would promise not to simmer long in resentment and hate against anyone if you were *certain* that by so doing you could lighten the burden on an ulcer.

You would take more frequent vacations if you were *certain* they would help keep you healthy.

You would take all of these precautions, especially if you had a bad family history of heart disease and were *certain* that good care of yourself would prevent an attack.

But how can you be certain if I (a doctor) am not

certain; nor is anyone else in the medical profession who is honest and open-minded about these problems.

Although a greater part of my life has been devoted to teaching the value of preventive medicine—directly, on the front lines of medical practice; and indirectly, by lecturing, writing articles and books on the subject of health preservation—I have come to believe that until recent theories of "life-endangerment" are proved **beyond a doubt,** that there is no valid, sensible reason for you to live too cautiously.

My philosophy is you only live once. *Yesterday is in the mind. Tomorrow is in the heart.* Today is your life. Learn to live it in full day by day or you die a little.

You can still have fun in living by following the ancient Greek rule: **nothing in excess.**

In some broad sense, we are all hypochondriacs. Job worries, health worries, survival worries make their insidious contributions to our chronic anxiety. You may worry about your health, another person about the imminence of the exploding bomb, and another about the welfare of his job and family. Job. Love. Security. Fear of illness and death. There are scores of variations. As a doctor, I have observed them in their many forms.

As a result, too many of us live half a life—or less—because our living is taken up with being scared.

As a doctor, my purpose is to un-frighten you. I propose to offer you a sensible health program. In many instances you will be happy to learn how to make a fair appraisal of yourself. Whether you are normally apprehensive or are abnormally worrisome, I hold out greater hope for you.

In the following chapters I shall discuss both the positive and negative aspects of the Ten Health Commandments I have enumerated earlier. By the time you have finished this book, I promise you that you will have become acutely aware that you only live once. And that you might as well go about making this one-way trip a success.

To help make this come true you must forget the Ten Health Commandments.

Stop being scared and remember—it's Your Life to Enjoy.

1

Thou shalt not
Take Cholesterol?

You don't have to stop living in order to live.

There are still some remaining pleasures you have the right to savor every day of your life. I know many people —doctors included—who have become so hipped on preventing illness that they have forgotten how to live.

For example, consider Dr. X. I saw him last about 10 years ago. I don't know whether he is alive or dead—but undoubtedly he believes that I must have been shuffled off many years ago. Dr. X. and I—as practicing internists and heart specialists—used to have many friendly disagreements. When I tried to form my medical judgments within an elastic framework of medical knowledge, my friend practiced and preached within an iron-bound, unyielding doctor-patient relationship.

If you had an ulcer or coronary disease and he caught you smoking, he would boot you out of the office and say, "Find yourself another doctor."

If you had high blood pressure and used a lot of salt: **ditto.**

If you dabbed a pat of butter on your toast: **ditto.**

If you took a drink before dinner: **ditto.**

I recall my friend as an almost mummified individual, with sunken cheeks and humorless countenance. In his case he practiced what he preached. He was cholesterol-conscious; exercise-conscious; a liquor and tobacco hater; a man who lived by mathematical formula. He could say truthfully, "Not only do as I say; you can do as I do."

No Definite Proof

About 15 years ago during a stay in Boston for a medical convention of the American College of Physicians we happened to meet in the lobby one morning and went into breakfast.

He ordered dry toast and tea. I had prunes with cream, wheat cakes, three tabs of butter, syrup, a slice of ham on the side, coffee with cream and sugar.

To say that Dr. X. regarded me with distaste is to put it mildly. His suffering became especially intense when I lit a cigarette—although I was careful not to blow smoke in his direction.

Pointedly, he said, "Going in to hear the paper on cholesterol this morning?".

I said I was. We sat together. I was not at all surprised to learn from the eminent speaker—and from other authorities who discussed the cholesterol problem—that we had no definite proof that a high cholesterol is the cause of hardening of the arteries (atherosclerosis) and therefore, of stroke, coronary artery disease, etc. Now, many years later, we still aren't sure. But Dr. X., and many others like him, believe it to be true beyond a doubt. As a result thousands of patients go through life discouraged and afraid. They are conscience-stricken even before they sit down to the table. Their heads are full of such terms as saturated fats, polyunsaturated fats, cholesterol and blood lipid levels.

Are You Too Cholesterol-Conscious?

How do you feel when you have ordered eggs and the two round, yellow eyes of eggs-sunnyside-up stare up at you? With all the talk about the dangers of saturated fats and cholesterol, don't you just visualize the sticky yellow stuff being transported by the blood to your coronary arteries and coating them with a thin layer of atherosclerosis which will surely do you in long before your time?

Butter, cream, eggs, fried foods, fatty meats, cookies, pies, cheese, cakes, ice cream—such saturated fats are supposed to be your mortal enemies. Is there any wonder that you eat in apprehension and feel like a grown-up kid caught with his hand in the cookie jar?

Oh, for the good old days when I was a kid and would run into the house just long enough to get a thick slice of bread, smeared with a heavy thickness of fresh butter, generously sprinkled with a layer of sugar and gulp a glass of milk.

But pity the kids of today! I've been reading some scientific papers which say that the treatment of atherosclerosis should begin much earlier! Saturated fats should be withheld from children, some doctors say. Whole milk, which they are used to drinking in abundance, may be the cause of most of the coronary disease and other troubles they bear in later years.

I'm sure my friend Dr. X. will vote Yea for that theory. My vote is Nay. If we are going to keep milk from children because of a *theory,* then that's going too far!

Difference of Opinion

A middle-aged college instructor said to me recently, "Although I have felt quite healthy otherwise, I have had a higher than normal cholesterol reading. I keep my weight down and am on a low cholesterol diet. A friend told me that you have discussed the cholesterol problem with him. I was happy to hear you told him that a high cholesterol doesn't always guarantee future trouble in the arteries. Did he misquote you?"

Not at all, I said. I remember telling him that too many people with readings above the normal 220-250 level live their lives steeped in trepidation, anxiety and actual fear. Although a high cholesterol reading is nothing to pass off lightly, neither is it something to sit down and cry about.

Perhaps we doctors often have been guilty of overstressing the connection between high cholesterol and atherosclerosis (the forerunner of coronary artery disease and stroke). It's only fair that we give you the other side, too. All you have been offered is depressing statistics. How about a change?

For example, in *Medical Digest* I read a condensation of an article which appeared in the *Canadian Medical*

Journal, written by Dr. J. C. Peterson and associates. They performed 191 autopsies on patients who had been permanently hospitalized with atherosclerosis; and who had routine serum cholesterol readings taken during their stay.

After carefully examining the cerebral, coronary and leg arteries they found that "analysis of these data did not show any significant relationship between the severity of the atherosclerosis and the level of serum cholesterol."

Here is Mr. M., a hard-working business man of 44. He has a blood cholesterol reading of 280. He has been on a low cholesterol diet and "worried sick" that he is a candidate for a coronary attack. He wants to know if there is anything new in the cholesterol problem.

There's nothing new. We are still as confused as ever regarding the real cause (or causes) of atherosclerosis.

Heredity, stress, over-or-under exercise, cigarette smoking, obesity, emotional binges, high blood cholesterol levels: such are among the prominent culprits we suspect, either singly, or in marauding groups.

High Cholesterol Not Always Troublesome

Mind you, I go along with most of the doctors who believe that a patient with a high cholesterol should reduce (if overweight) and cut down on the saturated fats (like butter, cream, fatty meats, etc.). But I am also aware that there's more to cholesterol excess than that. We know that large amounts of cholesterol are formed in the body irrespective of our diets.

I have seen many patients with high cholesterol readings go along into old age without having a coronary attack or cerebral thrombosis (stroke). A recent study bears out my personal experience in practice. Three Canadian doctors did a cholesterol study on 800 patients in an Ontario veterans' hospital. They made this notation: "The results lend little support to the contention that the severity of atherosclerosis is related to the level of serum cholesterol, except, perhaps, when it exceeds 300 milligrams per cent. In 58 cases in the age group 60-69 years, significant relationships between the level of serum cholesterol and the severity of disease were found only once in 40 statistical analyses."

I recall a husband and wife who came to me about ten years ago. Each had cholesterol readings in a range from 300 to 350. And each lived in fear of having coronary thrombosis. In spite of my repeated assurances, they would have these blood checkups at frequent intervals. Sometimes every week. They were typical "cholesterol-ophobes." I am happy to report that at a recent reunion they informed me that neither has had the attack they feared. The husband is now in his middle sixties, and his wife just turned 60.

Final Solution Still Eludes Us

In the *Connecticut State Medical Journal*, Dr. Lawrence W. Kinsell, Institute of Metabolic Research, Highland Ameda County Hospital, Oakland, California, wrote: "Of all the chemical compounds that are measured in clinical laboratories, there is none about which more has been written and about which less is understood than cholesterol." Since cholesterol is a normal essential part of the human body, "It is obvious that attempts to 'get rid of' this compound would be both unphysiological and impossible."

And Dr. W. Stanley Hartroft, of the Department of Pathology, Washington University Medical School, St. Louis—after rat studies at his school—has shown that the development of heart disease in an individual rat could not be predicted on the basis of its level of cholesterol.

Until we know more, I agree that patients should follow their doctors' advice regarding low cholesterol diets. But, as you see, the final answer evades us. And I believe that medical advice should be well-tempered and the edicts to patients delivered in a full measure of common sense.

Mass Anxiety About Cholesterol

Do you suffer from "cholesterol neurosis"? Does even the thought of butter or cream in your diet give you the shakes? Are you running to a medical laboratory every few weeks to have another test? Do you live in fear of a coronary attack? If so, don't think you are alone. Thousands are "running scared." The cause of this mass anxiety should be shouldered by Dr. X. and his cohorts.

Now please, don't think that I am underestimating the value of cholesterol readings—or the need to be on guard when your cholesterol is higher than normal. Our present knowledge about atherosclerosis and cholesterol certainly indicates that there is a relationship between the two— even if we are not quite sure what that is. Therefore, if there is a history of coronary disease in your family, you certainly should follow your doctor's instructions when he asks you to go on a low cholesterol diet.

All I am suggesting is that you do not become panicky about it all. Don't fear that the end is near. I think the following statistics may give you some assurance. In a recent study of 1,000 cases of proved coronary thrombosis reported by Dr. Teodoro Cesarman of the Instituto Nacional de Cardiologia in Mexico City, there was no significant elevation in serum cholesterol levels in most of the patients.

In other words, one is liable to have a coronary attack even when the reading is normal. You only borrow unnecessary trouble when you become too conscious about your cholesterol readings.

Listen to the provocative Dr. Sigmund L. Wilens in his book, *My Friends the Doctors,* when he was being treated for tuberculosis: "The new nurse's aide obviously believed that three eggs for breakfast constituted the last word in high living. So she insisted that I have this number every morning. I obliged her, and further indulged freely in other naughty foods that are supposed to bring on heart attacks, as did all the patients. Yet heart attacks on the tuberculosis wards of a hospital are practically unheard of."

Don't Tamper with Diets

An anxious father had what he thought was an awful problem. He said to me, "When my daughter was very young she would not eat eggs at all. Our pediatrician said she must have the eggs so he advised me to beat and strain a raw egg in a large glass of orange juice. She liked it so well that it became the major part of her breakfast. This has gone on for about 35 years. Now here's my question. Shall I advise her to stop? I've been reading and hearing that there is danger in cholesterol."

I told him to forget it. I said that I wished 100 per cent

of teenagers might have been brought up on a breakfast consisting at least of fresh orange juice and egg. How most of them grow up with the unbalanced (or often absent) diets they take is a mystery to me.

Not only are parents anxious about the diets of their children, they worry about themselves, their grandparents, their in-laws, their business associates, their other friends.

How often has a concerned daughter come to me and said, "I'm really worried about my mother. She eats enough butter and takes enough whole milk and cream to feed a family of six. Don't you think it's bad for her? Shouldn't I put a stop to it?"

"How old is your mother?"

"She's 80."

"Haven't you answered your own question?" I usually say. Sometimes the guileless parents are 79, 75 or in their early 70s. Unaware or unimpressed by the cholesterol statistics which bear evil tidings for those who indulge in exaggeration, these contented oldsters go on with the diet which has served them so well for many years.

Enjoy Your Breakfast

Listen to Mrs. X.:

"Is there a secret pact among doctors and health experts to make us all gibbering idiots? I am one of those vanishing Americans who enjoy breakfast. I don't mean a cup of coffee and a roll, either!

"For about 40 years I've had my bacon and eggs along with cereal, juice, hotcakes or whatever I might be in the mood for. But always bacon and eggs. One slice of toast is adequate since I only eat toast as long as the eggs last. I don't eat lunch but most always have a glass or two of milk, sometime between noon and 2 P.M.

"Since I have a hard-working husband I always prepare a good dinner. I am not a heavy eater at night but eat all I want. Well, now comes my problem, Dr. Steincrohn. I have been hearing and reading about low cholesterol diets. I'm doing all the wrong things! Is there any wonder I'm confused? For years we have been told by radio and TV that we never outgrow our need for milk; also that the older we get the more we need at least one egg a day.

"Woe is me! I wish the powers that be would get together and give *one* advice instead of giving us a lot of theories."

Mrs. X. is 48, is normal-weighted and has a normal cholesterol. Her husband is 53, has no family history of coronary disease, his blood pressure is normal and so is his weight. I told her that I saw no contra-indication to continuing her hot cakes, milk, bacon and eggs—and that her husband could join in the gustatory proceedings. I agree with her that as far as a good breakfast is concerned, there have been too many vanishing Americans.

Normal Cholesterol No Signal for Indiscretion

Mrs. Y. also has a problem with her husband. She said, "Sometimes I wonder if it is wise for some people to have a blood cholesterol taken. My husband is an example. Because his father and older brother died of coronary disease, he went to a laboratory for an examination. His blood cholesterol was normal. Since then he has kicked up his heels. He overeats, especially fats and fried foods. He also works too hard, drinks too much, and smokes at least one and one-half packs a day. He keeps saying he's different—that his cholesterol proves that he hasn't got anything to worry about. Don't you think I ought to bring him in so you can pound some good sense into him?"

She did and I talked to him. I said: "I consider your family history of coronary disease more important than your cholesterol readings. I am not saying that you are a sure candidate for a coronary attack because it seems 'to run in your family.' But I am saying that heredity is important.

"Your wife tells me that you are living high off the hog simply because a blood cholesterol reading was normal. Therefore, I want to warn you that a normal cholesterol is no guarantee against having a coronary attack. And conversely, that people with high blood cholesterol readings aren't necessarily sure candidates, either. Atherosclerosis, the forerunner of such attacks, can develop even when the blood is not overloaded with cholesterol."

Study of Baboons

Then I told him of an interesting study I had read recently. Dr. Henry C. McGill and his associates reported a study of the arteries of 163 baboons. In many there was evidence of atherosclerosis—the gradual closing off and damage to coats of arteries.

And what do baboons live on mostly? On fruits, berries and grains. Hardly any cholesterol in their diet. And how high was the blood cholesterol in these baboons? The average was 80 milligrams—which is quite low. Yet many had atherosclerosis.

"Mr. Y.," I said, "we are closer to baboons than you may realize. I hope this convinces you to slow down all around. Stop worrying your wife. I am not downgrading the importance of cholesterol readings; but they should not be the only consideration in the management of potential coronary disease and trouble in the brain arteries."

No Simple Answer

In this day and age, when heart disease is the recognized number one killer, it is not surprising to receive so many anxious requests on how to prevent coronary thrombosis.

Unfortunately, there is no simple answer. Doctors agree that there is much we are suspicious of, but so little we know definitely about its prevention.

For example, we recognize that atherosclerosis is the underlying cause for most coronary trouble. But what actually causes this deterioration in the walls of the arteries? What causes the lime salts and fatty acids, and cholesterol to infiltrate the walls and at last slowly fill up the bore of the artery and deprive the heart of its normal blood supply? And the brain of its normal supply? And the kidneys and all the rest of the organs?

Is tension a factor? Overexertion? Underexercise? Overweight? High cholesterol? Heredity? Tobacco? Who can say for certain?

I have known some people with high blood cholesterol readings who were tense, never exercised; whose father, mother and brothers had coronary disease; who oversmoked, overworked, overdrank—yet never came down with a coronary attack.

On the other hand, I have treated thin, relaxed, moderate workers of good habits and good heredity who got a coronary thrombosis in their middle forties. Why one and not the other? Just for the reasons I have been giving: we have not yet come up with the answer of atherosclerosis.

And yet many doctors treat patients as if we had the final solution. Recall what I told you about my friend Dr. X. who lives and acts the part of a man who is sure of the answer—in spite of so many conflicting opinions.

No Blanket Treatment

Personally, I cannot accept the pronouncements from some doctors that "if you don't get enough exercise, you'll get a coronary attack" or "if you don't relax a coronary will get you."

Mind you, in the light of our present knowledge I'm in favor of playing it as safe as we know how: less tension, less smoking and drinking, less overeating, less overexerting, moderate exercise, low cholesterol diet. But what I am against is blanket treatment of the entire community. I believe in treating each patient as an individual. That is why I allow some to smoke, some to stay overweight, some to work hard, some to be lazy, others to drink alcohol: because it is important to weigh severe restrictions in living against the opportunity to enjoy the few short years we have here.

I tell my colleagues: don't let's get too oracular until we are scientifically sure—until we really have the final answers.

Not all medical men agree on the need for change in

diet. For example, Dr. Frederick J. Stare of Harvard said
—as reported in *Science Digest* in April '57: "On the
basis of current information I do not believe it is justified
to recommend drastic changes in the quantity or type of
fat in the diet of the general population as a means of preventing coronary heart disease."

Dr. Stare contends there has been too much "sensationalism" entering the public and scientific discussion of hardening of the arteries and too much "public-finger-pointing"
at various dietary substances without sufficient research to
support accusations. There are many factors that might
contribute to the artery problem. He points out that sex
hormones, heredity and the extent of one's physical activity
also could be involved.

You may argue that opinion was written about six
years ago; but I think it still is true because of the subsequent plethora of information and misinformation.

For example, writing in the *Lancet,* a British medical
periodical, Drs. M. F. Oliver and G. S. Boyd said that
in men with coronary heart disease, continued reduction
of serum lipids (cholesterol, etc.) does not appear to reduce the incidence of subsequent myocardial infarction
(coronary attack).

Is the evidence I have been slowly piling up for you
refreshingly reassuring, or are you wondering: "What
gives with this fellow? He's a doctor, isn't he? Then why
is he running down the cholesterol theory?"

Healthy Man Need Not Live Scared

If you believe that, there's either something wrong with
my "sending" station or too much static on your "re-

ceiving" end. All I have been trying to do is give you the other side of the picture. The choice is yours, to believe or disbelieve the present cholesterol theory. And the choice isn't simple.

Any patient who comes to me with a very high cholesterol, obesity, high blood pressure, changes in his electrocardiograms and other evidence of trouble would certainly receive this advice: "Better take off some weight, limit your intake of saturated fats"—among other suggestions.

However, if an apparently healthy man of 40 came in wondering if he should cut down on his usual food intake, I would say, "I'll let you know in a few days."

I'd then take a complete personal history, take cholesterol readings, electrocardiograms, do a physical, take x-rays and any other laboratory tests that were indicated. If he were a really healthy man I'd say: "Forget you ever heard the word cholesterol. As long as you keep your weight within normal bounds there's no reason why you have to stop having milk, cheeses, steaks, ice cream sundaes and all the rest of the foods you like."

What "gives" with me? I have a lot of distinguished company. For instance, sit at the feet of Arthur Grollman, M.D., professor and chairman of the Department of Experimental Medicine at the University of Texas Southwestern Medical School: "We really should avoid giving patients the impression that cholesterol alone is the answer to the problem of atherosclerosis. Clearly it is not. We do not need to encourage the prevailing air of panic about cholesterol."

He said—and I and others have been also saying it for years—that medical men should urge people to avoid excesses of fats, but people should be urged to avoid ex-

cesses of anything else. And certainly it is good sense to re-
strict fats in people who are overweight and whose blood
cholesterol levels are high.

Nevertheless, he said: "All the facts about cholesterol
and atherosclerosis are not in yet. Until they are, we can
help our patients most just by encouraging ordinary dis-
cretion."

Are you beginning to feel better? Can you now look
straight into the benign, yellow eyes of your poached eggs
every morning? Or, are you a die-hard? Are you on my
friend Dr. X.'s side? Do you prefer to live the Spartan
life?

Would You Want to Live Like This Man?

If so, perhaps you will be interested in the following,
which helps illustrate my point. It was written by Dale
Groom, M.D., of Charleston, South Carolina. It appeared
in the *Annals of Internal Medicine* and is called, "Population Studies of Atherosclerosis." In a footnote to his
article, Dr. Groom has written the "Thumbnail Sketch of
the Man Least Likely to Have Coronary Disease." It goes
like this:

"An effeminate municipal worker or embalmer,
Completely lacking in physical and mental alertness and
    without drive, ambition or competitive spirit who has
    never attempted to meet a deadline of any kind.
A man with poor appetite, subsisting on fruit
    and vegetables laced with corn and whale oils,
Detesting tobacco,
Spurning ownership of radio, TV, or motor car,
With full head of hair and

Scrawny and non-athletic in appearance,
Yet constantly straining his puny muscles by
    exercise;
Low in income, B.P., blood sugar, uric acid and
    cholesterol,
Who has been taking nicotinic acid, pyridoxine,
    and long term anticoagulant therapy
Ever since his prophylactic castration."

Would you live this kind of life to prevent coronary disease? Even if it were foolproof and guaranteed to keep the inner coat of your arteries glistening as smooth as satin? I suppose there are exceptions among you, but many will think, "Live like that and then get hit by a car while on the way to the store to buy some corn oil? Not for me!"

Sensible Lawyer

Listen to my friend, a 45-year-old trial lawyer, who has reacted with more than ordinary vehemence to the nation-wide cholesterol phobia:

"I'm not falling for all this hysteria about the dangers of cholesterol. In my job decisions are made on incontestable evidence. The just and true verdict depends upon un-disputed facts. From what I have heard and read about this problem I would hesitate to take on the prosecution of cholesterol in court as an assassin beyond doubt. There are too many ifs and buts; too much circumstantial evidence.

"You may think I'm some kind of peculiar guy, but I refuse to surrender to mass fear. I feel fine. A recent phys-

ical shows that I'm OK. Why should I worry? I am re-
duced to utter boredom when I hear my friends talk about
reducing diets, saturated and non-saturated fats.

"When I sit down to dinner I have a steak with all the
fixings. If I feel like having pie à la mode for dessert, I
do so with a clear conscience. I take cream in my coffee,
butter on my potatoes and have two eggs every morning
for breakfast. Yet, I'm sensible enough to cut down on
calories if I feel my weight may be going up.

"I have an associate who lives in fear. He won't join me
in a beer because it is fattening—yet he is as skinny as a
rail. He lives on skim milk, sauerkraut juice, chicken, fish
and dry toast. I can't go out to eat with him because
watching him nibble fearfully at his food—if you call it
that—makes me sick. And I suppose that he feels the
same when he watches me.

"He keeps warning me that eating raw onions will ruin
my stomach; that fats will clog my arteries; that too much
salt will raise my blood pressure; that I ought to go in
every few weeks to have a cholesterol reading.

"But I tell him to stop worrying about me and begin
worrying about himself. About beginning to live a little,
I mean. When I think of how many precious hours and
days he—and so many others—waste it makes me feel ill.
Scrounging along, half-living in fear of what **might** happen
is certainly no way to take advantage of God's goodness
in giving us life and the means to enjoy it."

Ah! To hear and see at least one person in these
darkened days of despair who lives with gusto and without
fear. And why not? A recent overhaul shows that his
weight, blood pressure, blood cholesterol, heart and all the
rest are normal. He takes advantage of the good news.

Too many, equally well, are waiting around for something bad to happen. They live dismal, frightened lives. How about you?

Summary of Chapter

1. Don't stop living in order to live.
2. **We still have no definite proof that a high cholesterol causes atherosclerosis,** and therefore, stroke or coronary disease.
3. Don't be stared into submission by the two yellow eyes of eggs sunny-side-up.
4. Saturated fats are not the mortal enemies of everyone.
5. There is no definite relation between the height of cholesterol and the severity of atherosclerosis.
6. In atherosclerosis, it is true that heredity, stress, over-or-under-exertion, smoking, obesity, high blood pressure and emotional binges are considerations as important as the cholesterol level.
7. A normal cholesterol reading is no guarantee against having a stroke or coronary thrombosis. Conversely, a high reading doesn't mean that you are a sure candidate.
8. Recall Dr. Lawrence W. Kinsell's statement: "Of all the chemical compounds that are measured in clinical laboratories, there is none about which more has been written and about which less is understood than cholesterol."
9. Take a long, impartial look at yourself: do you suffer unnecessarily from "cholesterol neurosis"?
10. There is no scientific basis for keeping milk from youngsters.

11. Don't try to change the "bad habits" of those who have already reached their seventies or eighties.

12. Even baboons—who live mostly on fruits, berries and grains—get atherosclerosis.

13. Remember the contention of Dr. Frederick J. Stare of Harvard that there is too much "sensationalism" entering the public and scientific discussion of hardening of the arteries.

14. Also, the statement of Arthur Grollman, M.D.: "We do not need to encourage the prevailing air of panic about cholesterol. All the facts about cholesterol are not in yet."

15. Turn again to Dr. Dale Groom's amusing, yet ironic description of the man least likely to get coronary disease. Would you care to live like that man?

16. "The role of cholesterol in heart and artery disease has not been established," says the Food and Drug Administration.

17. Reread the entire chapter. It will be worth the trouble. For the first time in many months you will then be able to sit down with full enjoyment to a breakfast of bacon and eggs, or to a steak dinner with all the "fixin's"—without any nagging anxieties to disturb your appetite.

The FIRST Commandment: Thou Shalt Not Take Cholesterol

Forget it IF:

1. You are 70 or over
2. Your weight is normal and/or
3. Your blood pressure is normal and/or
4. Your physical examination and electrocardiograms are normal and/or
5. Your blood sugar is normal and/or
6. You have good heredity.

NOTE:

Being healthy, don't live as if you are sick. Excluding cholesterol is no guarantee for the future. Why sacrifice the present? Dare to live without fear of fried foods, fatty foods, the high cholesterol foods.

Remember it IF:

1. You are more than 20 pounds overweight and/or
2. Your blood pressure is elevated and/or
3. You have had an attack of coronary thrombosis or a stroke and/or
4. You have angina pectoris and/or
5. You have diabetes and/or
6. Your cholesterol readings remain above normal and/or
7. Your heart is enlarged and there are specific changes in your electrocardiograms.
8. Your family history unveils cases of stroke or coronary diseases; high blood pressure or diabetes.

The FIRST Commandment: Thou Shalt Not Take Cholesterol *(Continued)*

NOTE:

If you have any condition which suggests the need for taking less cholesterol, remind yourself that other restrictions may be even more important: Don't overeat. Don't overwork. Don't be tense. Don't overexercise. Don't take tobacco or alcohol.

2

Thou shalt not
Be Lazy?

You can rest in the hammock and still keep fit.

An accusation which brings many of us shame and degradation is the term "lazy." Acutely, we resent being thrown into that category; as if we were cast into a cell filled with groveling, indolent creatures.

"Me lazy! Whatever gave you that idea?" And then if you are weak-willed, you deliberately set out to prove that you haven't got a lazy bone in your body.

Although it hurts—both physically and emotionally—you go about being active. You overcome your innate distaste for exertion. You walk miles, you bowl, play tennis or golf (or both), you go in for gymnastics.

All the while you hate it. You'd prefer lying down somewhere just doing nothing. But the designation "lazy" grates on you.

Man Who Killed Himself

I recall the sad case of a man of about 45 who actually killed himself while trying to prove that he wasn't lazy. I had taken care of Mr. J., a successful salesman for a large firm, for many years. I knew him as both friend and patient.

Until he was in his early forties he was an active, resourceful fellow who delighted in physical exertion. He played 18 holes of golf every Sunday—rain or shine. He played tennis with his teenaged youngsters. He never just sat around the house. "Let's do something" was his watchword. He mowed the lawn, painted the house, and puttered around all the time. His wife used to say, "The trouble with Fred is that he can't sit still. I wish you could give him something to slow him up a little."

But then Nature took a hand. He came to me one morning complaining of a smothering feeling in his chest when he walked.

"I can't understand it," he said. "Lately I can't walk more than a block before I have to stop and rest. When the pain goes away in a few minutes, I go on again as if nothing happened."

Fred Had Angina

His physical and electrocardiographic examinations were negative—as they often are in patients who have angina pectoris. (Patients who have chest pain on exertion because of diseased coronary arteries.) Nevertheless, I prescribed some nitroglycerin. He told me that when he put a tablet under his tongue that the pain disappeared as if by magic.

Later, "exercise" electrocardiograms showed changes indicative of coronary disease. His attacks became more frequent. I told him he had angina and mapped out a new way of life for him. I informed his wife that I expected him to slow down and curtail some of his physical activities. She seemed to understand; but soon forgot.

As his chest discomforts became more frequent, this once active man gradually put on the brakes. He gave up tennis. He played only five or nine holes of golf on weekends. Instead of fussing around the house, he would lie around on Sunday recharging his battery so he could go out and see his customers during the week. But being lazy wasn't easy.

Frustrated and Unhappy

One day he came to me utterly confused and frustrated. He said, "What bothers me more than the pains I get is the attitude of my wife and children. On weekends, when I am lying in the hammock reading, or sitting in a rocker just thinking of what a tough break it is for an active man to have to slow up so much—to top it all I feel conscience-stricken.

"My wife will say, 'Well, if you won't take a hand in the lawn-mowing, I guess I'll have to do it myself.' Or my son will say, 'I don't suppose there's any use asking you to play some tennis'— as if I was a lazy lout. Perhaps I don't complain to them enough. I ought to tell them that these chest pains are bothering me more and more.

"For example, the other day after work—and I've had to cut down on my customer calls—my wife asked me to help her hang some pictures. I got up on a ladder, and will you believe it I almost died while I was up there. Just having to raise my hands above my head and pound in a few tacks almost did me in. I'm sure I was pale and sweaty when I finished; either she didn't notice it or thought I was putting on an act. That I resented being disturbed.

Tragedy

"Sometimes I wish I was a dog. When they're sick they can crawl away to some corner and suffer undisturbed. How is it possible for a man's family to forget that when he was healthy, he was an active normal man? What is there about being lazy that's so terrible even if you're not sick? People make you feel that you're the lowest of the low if you have no desire to move your muscles around."

I told him to charge it up to misunderstanding, not actual cruelty. I said I would call his wife and tell her that he was sick, not lazy. I did, but wondered from our conversation, if she didn't believe that Fred and I were in cahoots.

Two weeks later, in weather fit neither for man nor bear, they picked him off the sidewalk in front of his house. He had died while shoveling snow. I will never know if his family goaded him into these unnatural exertions, or if he did it on his own to "prove he wasn't lazy."

We Are Made From Many Molds

Human beings come in all shapes, forms and inclinations. You can't change the color of a man's eyes (except by contact lenses); or make a 6-footer out of a five-by-five; or convert a person who has an actual aversion to physical activity into a physical culture addict. I keep reminding people to remember this. It will promote better understanding of our fellows. It will cut down on the number of persons who are always trying to convert the naturally inactive individual into a dynamo.

I have made special note of this: lazy people are content to be lazy without trying to influence others to partake of the pleasures of the rocking chair and hammock; but exercise-conscious persons are forever trying to make converts to their way of life.

Thomas Hardy, the English novelist, said: "The man who writes stands up to be shot at."

You don't have to dig too far down into that sentence to recognize what he meant. For instance, the doctor who expresses medical opinions easily available to millions of readers, is an inviting target for pot shots from persons who disagree (laymen and doctors alike). He gets letters of appreciation; but also his share of letters of mild or bitter disagreement.

But I hope to have Hardy's good fortune: although he stood up in full view, no barrage from a discontented reader ever found a vital spot. He lived to be 86 years old.

Can't Please All Readers

Any number of subjects will especially irk readers. For example, if I write that I do not advise **everybody** to stop smoking (even though I have emphasized that many should stop) I am sure to get protesting letters against this "bad medical advice."

If I mention that alcohol is occasionally of value in medical treatment, the arrows whiz by thick and dangerously close. The readers overlook and skip my exclamatory sentences which emphasize the dangers inherent in chronic alcoholism. All they remember is that I am advocating we become a nation of topers.

But those well-meant recriminations are as nothing compared to what I have been hearing for years in answer to my convictions against exercise. From all over this shrinking globe I have been getting shot at by the arrows of exercise-addicts and zealots.

If they could lay hands on me they would throw away their arrows and tear me apart with their superbly muscled arms. Although I have never held up a bank, they call me Public Enemy Number One. Simply because I had the temerity over 20 years ago to write a book—and since, many articles for national magazines—saying that **you don't have to exercise!**

What long memories these people have. And, frankly, I am glad of it. I relish their disaffection; especially since the arrows they sling are not really poison-dipped.

Hard Lesson

For years I have been writing that over-exercise can kill you. And I write about it again now because I have just heard that another one of my doctor friends (who should have known better) was recently carried off the tennis courts with a "coronary." When he recovers I know I shall have another convert—although I hate to get them in this manner. (I can't talk people into being on my side; it seems they need to be in a near-tragedy first.)

Until now my friend has disagreed that exercise will hurt the normal heart. What needs emphasizing again, however, is this: when you go out on a tennis court or engage in 36 holes of golf on a weekend, are you sure that your above-40 heart is normal?

The odds are at least ten to one that you don't know. Because it is at least ten to one that you go to your doctor only when you are sick. Not before! The majority of people do not go in for yearly physical checkups. And that is the gist of it all. You gamble with your life when you don't know. Over-exercise is poison for the sick heart if taken in large doses.

Is or Isn't Your Heart Normal?

I found some interesting statistics written by Dr. Louis Dublin in his book *The Facts of Life:* "It is a common but erroneous belief that strenuous physical activity can damage the heart. The healthy heart can stand almost any physical activity without being impaired. However, over-exertion can prove fatal to the person with the diseased heart. Common examples are persons who die suddenly while playing tennis or running after trains. This is not to say the cardiacs should avoid all exercise. They should, however, adjust their activity according to their personal limitations."

Therefore, the problem boils down to one of early recognition. Do you—or don't you—have a normal heart? If you do you may exercise moderately. If you don't, you may kill yourself. In spite of these definitive statements, I expect to continue to be a target (as in the past) for "exercise-conscious" readers.

They will be saying, "He said exercise is bad for the heart."

Nevertheless, I hope that so many of you will be on my side, that these dissenters will continue to be a minority group. Some day—and I hope it's soon—they, too, will wake up to the need for giving their middle-aged heart a break before it breaks them.

According to a story I read in the paper quite a few years ago, Danny Thomas, comedian, sustained a broken ankle. Not, mind you, while cavorting around the stage or while making a film. It seems a few college boys were visiting his daughter Margaret, 18, and got up a basketball game in the Thomas yard. You can guess the rest. The then 42-year "old man" must have begged to get into the game. He'd show these modern youngsters now the game really should be played. I think that Danny's pride must have hurt him more than his ankle when they carried him off.

I Was a Victim Myself

I speak from experience. At the age of 40—right after publication of my exercise book warning those over 40 to refrain from overexertion—I was anxious to get into a softball game which was to be played on a farm in Vermont. After cajoling and begging the captain of one of the teams, Robert Frost, to let me play he at last agreed. He said something to the effect: "This is a dangerous game for people in their forties." He himself was in his sixties at the time.

During my first turn at bat, I slipped on my way to first base—and was carried off the field with the world's finest charley horse. On crutches for a few weeks afterwards, my discomfort was certainly not eased by seeing the knowing twinkle in the wonderful eyes of Robert Frost and of my erstwhile "over forty" team-mates.

I tell you this experience so you will know that I am as frail and open to temptation to overexercise as any other human being.

We people over forty just can't seem to accept the fact that we aren't good enough to compete with youngsters—or even with those in our own age group—where sudden bursts of physical activity are needed. Time after time we are thrown for a loss by children many years our juniors. I recall that when she was three years old, Rocky Marciano's daughter threw him, and put him into a hospital with a slipped disc!

Two Interesting Cases

I remember a 42-year-old woman who prided herself upon her youthfulness and slim figure. One day she got into a basketball game at a gymnasium with some teenagers. In rushing for the ball she misjudged and ran head-on into a concrete wall.

Fortunately, all she got was a concussion—but she suffered from headaches for years. She said, "What a dope! Imagine me trying to prove to myself—and perhaps to those kids—that I have a special contract with Father Time to remain young forever. Better warn your middle-aged patients to behave, doctor, or they'll be getting into worse trouble than I have."

Years ago I worked in a medical clinic with a fine medical man of about 45. He was leaving that afternoon, he said, for some skiing. "Aren't you too old to be taking that up now?" I said.

"Who, me?" he said.

Three days later they brought him back with a broken thigh. I visited him. He smiled and said: "No fool like an old fool—especially when the old fool is a doctor who should know better."

My orthopedic friends tell me that a good part of their time is taken up in treating "silly injuries" in older persons that shouldn't have happened. It's one thing to engage in moderate exercise if you enjoy it; it's something else to take on competitive sports and risk your head and heart. Or back—in doing the twist.

Don't Be a Middle-Aged Athlete

I have seen too much unnecessary misery of this kind. Therefore, at the risk of enraging my "middle-aged athlete friends," I warn you again.

If you insist on tennis, never play singles with a youngster. Play doubles with those in your own age group. As regards golf, better not try to get in 36 holes a day. Nine holes is preferable. Or eighteen, with a long rest in between the nines.

I am not against all exercise. You may bowl, garden, walk, or take other exertions provided they are in moderation. As for myself, I prefer to take mine in a rocking chair.

At this time it is only fair that you know to what form of existence I am addicted: to the physically lazy and indolent, or to the physically active. I am "lazy" yet consider myself a hard worker. It is possible to work sitting down. And bearing on what I have just said, I hope you won't think I am trying to influence you to become physically lazy.

What I am saying on the subject bears upon my reflection after observation of patients and others over a period of many years. I have tried to look at the problem —and problem it is—with cold, scientific detachment. So please, don't cast aside my observations as those made by a lazy man who is trying to "make you over." As I said, lazy people are notorious for minding their own business and letting others live their own lives in their own way.

You Don't Have to Exercise

Quite a number of years ago I wrote a book called: *You Don't Have to Exercise (Rest Begins at Forty).* After careful observation of the well and the sick in the interim, I have found little to change my opinion that exercise is not necessary for good health. I adhere to it in spite of the epidemic-like wave of enthusiasm that is sweeping the United States; in spite of the edicts from the White House that we must exercise and become more active to keep fit and make our country strong.

I believe in the need for exercise to promote fitness in young children, adolescents, and in college students. They need a good base and framework. But comes 40 and I think that overexertion should be taken in measured and careful doses—and not as a general panacea for every-one—regardless of physical ability or inclination.

He Couldn't Sit Still

I recall a prominent newspaper editor who spent every spare hour on the tennis courts, in the gym, or otherwise devising ways to overcome inertia. He wouldn't be "caught dead in a chair" unless he could help it. He never sat down for lunch. A soft drink and a sandwich, while stand-ing at a drugstore counter, was his five-minute stopover while on the way to the gymnasium to work out in a hand-ball game or run around the track. You could see that he was devoted to the ideal of physical fitness.

Although he had the choice of two cars to take him to work every morning and bring him home in the evening, he preferred to walk. I would wave to him as I passed on my way to the hospital. Long ago I had learned that inviting him for a lift was silly. His curt "thanks" carried with it a note of derision as you sped on in your car.

On occasion I had the chance to talk to this highly cerebral man about exercise. I would not bring up the subject because, as I mentioned earlier, his top-spinning gyrations never bothered me. Live and let live has been my motto. Why give him unasked advice or try to change him?

Once, at a cocktail party, we gravitated to a quiet corner and he began a dissertation on physical fitness.

"Here, feel this," he said, offering me his right biceps. "Not bad for a 46-year-old whose work keeps him at a desk all day."

I felt the rock-like protuberance under his coat sleeve and said, "H-m-m."

"You don't seem impressed," he said.

"I didn't think you were trying to impress me."

"To tell you the truth, I was," he said. "I understand that you're an exponent of the lazy life. I don't understand how a doctor like you can advise people that they don't have to exercise to keep well. Take me for example. I'd die if I couldn't take a good bit of exercise every day. Would you tell me to stop?"

I told him that there were many ifs and buts, many pros and cons.

"Come now," he said. "Let's not evade the issue. Would you tell me to quit?"

"All right," I said. "Let me dispose of the pros and cons quickly. I'm *for* your taking exercise every day if you like it (which you seem to do) and if you are physically able to take the added exertions. In other words, I'm supposing—not being your doctor—that your heart, blood pressure and the rest are in good condition.

"You see I'm not all bad. I believe that people who like exercise and are able to take it may continue. However, I'm *against* your unnatural gyrations if you are not physically able to take them safely."

"But I am ok physically," he said. "Just had a physical last week. I've been told that my heart's perfect."

"Remember," I said, "you brought this up. I didn't. So you'll have to suffer the discomfort of listening to a lecture. Once you get me started on exercise, I go along like the babbling brook."

"Go along, I'm game," he said.

I pounded his ears for at least a half hour. He took it like a good sport. I knew I couldn't influence him to change; and I didn't care if he did or didn't. But at least he heard me out.

In essence, here is what I told him.

Old Heart Not Like Young Heart

Many a middle-aged man who gets the good news from his doctor that his heart is all right immediately translates this verdict into one of super-optimistic connotations. He can now climb mountains, play tennis singles with teen-agers, play 36 holes of golf on a weekend, get up a good sweat in handball—in fact engage in any activities a youngster takes in stride. That's just where trouble can come winging in noiselessly.

If you are past forty remember that your normal heart is no match for a youngster's. It may be normal for you, and the things you should sensibly limit yourself to as age progresses; but if you should try to match his present pace with your "normal" heart you would break down early. Keep remembering the basic difference between what is normal for one age and another.

And your heart is not the only organ to consider. I think the state of your arterial tree is even more important. No matter how well you have taken care of yourself over the years, you can be sure that the inner coats of your arteries are showing evidence of the wear and tear.

Doesn't it make sense to take it easier on tires that have gone 20-30,000 miles? What would you think of a man who sped unconcernedly along at 70 miles an hour? Would you like to be sitting next to him as he raced his engine on such flimsy and blow-out susceptible rubber? Chances are that you'd never ride with him again—unless he got some new tires. Remember the old rubber in your inner tubes—although normal in the sense that you've never had a puncture—is liable to rip under pressure. Older arteries are that way, too. You may not have had a coronary thrombosis to warn you of a weakness in the nutrient-structure of your heart (just as the tires are normal in that they haven't had a blow out) but who's to say if and when one was in the offing. And would you rather be in a car going at ten miles an hour and blow a tire or at seventy? Would you rather treat your arteries with respect or tempt fate by putting them under pressure and keeping it on day after day with needless exertions?

Exertion and Coronary Thrombosis

Some doctors will tell you that you can get a coronary thrombosis while sitting or lying down. Exertion, they say, has nothing to do with it. It's true that many attacks occur while resting. But I do not agree with those who say that exertion can't bring on an attack.

On July 4, 1962 I read this disturbing report written by the Associated Press—dateline, Toronto, Canada:

"Heart attacks killed five Shriners Tuesday, casting a pall over thousands of their lodge brothers in the brassy opening of the 88th North American Shriner's Convention.

"Three of the victims collapsed in a mammoth parade that snaked through the center of Toronto for more than five hours. The two others died in their hotel rooms in the early morning. The temperature was a relatively mild 77 degrees."

Nowhere was there mention of "parade watchers" coming down with fatal attacks. With repeated evidence that excitement and overexertion bring on coronary attacks, some doctors still will not admit it.

It is not likely you will get an attack *watching* someone shoveling snow. I have made it a practice of asking my coronary thrombosis patients—who may have had their attack while resting—what they were doing in the day or two before the attack. Or, in the few weeks or months before. Invariably, there is a history of overexertion or strain.

The most severe attack with recovery I ever saw occurred in a man who admitted to me later (he knew he had angina) that he had rolled four heavy trash cans out to the curb during subzero weather. He was surprised that he "got away with such foolishness," he told me. Not until midnight (seven hours later) did he have the crushing pains of coronary thrombosis. If I hadn't asked, here would be another patient who had an attack while at rest.

Universal Cry: Fitness!

What is the actual need for people over 40 to be so physically fit? To have strong muscles, be able to run around the block or walk ten miles a day without effort? I can see no practical need for such fitness. "Let's keep our nation fit" is the universal cry you hear now. Why, I ask, other than our youngsters?

We have come a long way since our ancestral cave dwellers or other uncivilized counterparts. They needed to be fit from the neck down to survive. Whatever their age, a chance meeting with a wild animal (human or otherwise) was a challenge they had to be able to overcome—or perish. To feed and clothe their wives and offspring they needed to be sufficiently strong to bring down dangerous game.

20th-Century Fitness

How about now? What does it take other than thumb-pressure to open the ice-box or freezer? Our homes are heated in the winter and air-cooled during the summer. We have a standing army of police and firemen to protect us. Every want and desire can be had for moderate payment. The telephone is always at hand to insure human contact and orders for creature comforts.

Fit? Of course we have to be fit. But only from the neck up! Cerebral fitness is what gives many the protection and comforts our untamed and less intelligent ancestors fought and bled for.

Here are some points to remember. Fitness doesn't cure constipation. Fitness doesn't prevent serious disease. Fitness doesn't guarantee that you won't get a heart attack. It nas not been proved—in spite of what you hear—that the lazy man is more likely to get a coronary thrombosis than the one who is active. In fact, I think it's the other way around.

Show me the man who lives a leisurely life but keeps

his weight within normal limits; who keeps his emotions under control; who is not overly ambitious; who takes frequent vacations and knows how to laugh and relax; who has developed a sensible philosophy of life; whose habits are moderate and not taxing: and I'll wager on him in the health-race against the overactive physical culture enthusiast who is throwing away his precious heart beats in unnecessary exercise.

You Get More Exercise Than You Realize

However lazy you are, you get more exercise than you realize. The man who says he does nothing but sit at a desk all day, gets a bigger daily workout than he realizes. Getting up to go to the water cooler gives him exercise. Going out for his numerous coffee breaks gives him exercise. Walking into the supervisor's office to give and receive reports gives him exercise. Mowing the lawn gives him exercise. So does walking the dog. Going to the corner store for cigarettes does the same. Taking off his shoes and trousers. Pulling on his pajamas. Getting into a heavy overcoat during the winter. Bringing the fork to his mouth while eating. Sitting back in his chair for a big belly laugh at some joke. Rising to his feet during a football game to give vent to his emotions and pound his friend on the back. Add them up—these and hundreds more—and you will realize that few of us live like the tortoise (who, incidentally, lives to a good old age— lazy as he is).

Test of Laziness

I have great respect for the lazy people in this world. The physically lazy, that is. I'm sure the **wheel** was invented by a lazy man. Some of the world's greatest giant steps have been taken by people who hated to take actual physical steps.

If you are lazy, don't be openly boastful and prideful of it. I doubt that you will be. But have that inner satisfaction that we lazy fellows have when we watch the people who can't sit still go off on bicycle-jaunts, stairclimbs, muscle contortions before an open window, rowing machine exertions—and the hundreds of other ways devised by people who can't sit still to keep others from doing the same.

You are truly lazy if you can lie in your hammock with a book and look unconcernedly on some of your companions who are passing you with lifted eyebrows and derisive countenances—clutching their rackets and golf clubs. If you can remain one hundred per cent consciencefree under such circumstances; if you don't flinch at the actual accusation "lazy lout"—then you are one of us.

You are truly lazy if you actually ache as you watch someone with a green thumb working for hours in a garden or on the lawn—bending, perspiring, twisting, pulling, digging. But that doesn't make you a moron, unfit physically and mentally, to do your part as an American citizen. We aren't unpatriotic just because we don't thrash our muscles and whip ourselves into a daily burst of extra contortions.

Reactions to Article

Some years ago I wrote an article on the subject of exercise for *The Saturday Evening Post*. They called it *Learn to be Lazy*. From all over the United States I received letters and cards either calling me a lazy dolt or a matchless man of good sense. The former correspondents were the physical culturists; the latter were, of course, the large brigade of lazy people who believe in conserving their energies.

I recall that one man wrote: "I've just had a birthday. I celebrate every year by taking a swim in our lake. When I was forty I swam half a mile; when fifty, a mile; when sixty a mile and a half. I was seventy yesterday and took off for two miles. How about that?"

"Fine," I answered. "Keep up the good work. I'm really waiting to hear about your three-mile swim."

And there was the card from an 80-year-old who said, "Read your article on how to be lazy. It was fine but I really didn't need to read it. I'm relaxing here celebrating my birthday by sitting in my rocking chair watching everybody run around and fuss. I've been lazy all my life. I wouldn't bend over to pick up a ten-dollar bill if it was in front of my nose. How about that?"

I answered him, too. And I wondered—but not for long—that both letters had ended the same way: "How about that?" It proved to me what I have been saying right along: that the world is made up of all kinds of people, who sometimes know what's better for them than doctors or other people do.

Bill Brown, famous trainer, used to say: "It isn't the

it to homemaker.) I wish people would consider the three physical types we fall into: endomorphs, mesomorphs and ectomorphs. They should read "Varieties of Physique," by Dr. William H. Sheldon and the "Varieties of Temperament" by the same doctor. Also in Gesell Institute's *Child Behavior*, on pages 54-65, there is interesting information about the different types which, I am sure, will help all parents and physical educators to understand children and themselves, too. In these pages you will readily understand why some people *love* exercise and football and baseball etc. while others would rather watch from the sidelines as spectators—*and not be forced* to participate in games for which their bodies are not inclined. Each type has different drives, different responses, different interests. The mesomorph loves exercise and activity. The ectomorph shrinks from such activity. The endomorph loves comfort and relaxation. So I say let the mesomorphs and other types with leanings toward mesomorphy do all the strenuous exercise, and for heaven's sake let us ectomorphs and endomorphs relax on the sidelines as our body structures intended us to do. It is torture to engage in sports your body was not built for."

Whereas one human being may find it difficult to change one's inclinations from the lazy to the active life—and vice versa—Nature can accomplish the transformation so gently that you may not be aware of the change until you examine yourself carefully.

I Wasn't Born Lazy

I speak from personal experience. Many people who recognize in me an anti-exercise demon, believe that I must have been born lazy. Not true. As a youngster and a Boy Scout I delighted in every variation of physical exertion. I liked camping and roughing it. Enjoyed the long hikes and other tiring activities. I used to take long bike trips with some of my more enthusiastic cohorts. As I grew older I boxed and played baseball. I went out for track and played one year of college football.

When I began the practice of medicine I was in charge of a medical clinic where I was due every morning at 8:30. Nevertheless, I got up early at least three mornings a week to give me time to get in nine holes of golf before clinic. Later on in practice I used to make time to play at least nine holes a day three times a week at a golf club. Often, a half dozen of us doctors would meet during lunch hour to bowl a few strings.

Then came forty. Without realizing it at the time—and not because I had become mesmerized by the numerals 40 —I began to lose inclination to exert unnecessarily. The bowling sessions stopped. My golf gradually went down to once a week; then a game every few months. Within a few years I put away my clubs because I had lost all desire to play. (I know a lawyer friend of mine who will swear that I gave up golf because of missing a crucial one-foot putt on the 18th hole during a foursome battle.) In the last ten years I have played about three times. Try as I might, I could not relight the spark. Even now it's difficult to believe that I used to be the fellow who couldn't wait for the snows to melt so I could play; who used to practice putting into a cup on the living room floor.

Yet there are so many others who are diametrically opposite. As youngsters they were not exercise-minded. Now they have become fishing addicts or golf-nuts. They are always rushing through business to play a game or catch some fish. Others have become big-biceps-minded.

They have gone in for body-building at the age of 40 or 50—or older.

I call them middle-aged athletes. Either they're trying to prove something to themselves or they are trying to impress others. One man will attempt to prove he isn't growing old by having an extra-marital affair; another by trying to show off his muscles.

President Looks Comfortable in Rocking Chair

I tell these people to go ahead in moderation—if they really like to exert physically. I'm sure all don't. There are those who fall into line like sheep because they've heard that "exercise is good for you." That it's a "must."

President Kennedy, active most of his life, sounded the bugle for physical fitness. Many rush in to rally round the flag whether they like exercise or not. Yet, disabled by a distressing back disorder, I note that the President didn't look too uncomfortable as he sat in his rocking chair. Young as he was, he didn't look too incongruous in this most respectable and sensible article of furniture. In fact, I suspect that he was beginning to like a measure of physical relaxation.

Be true to your nature and basic inclinations.

Are you physically lazy? Don't be ashamed of it. You can hold your head as high as the fellow who is always throwing his muscles, bones and joints around. There's no special honor in belonging to the cult of the physically active. Nor is there any added guarantee of healthfulness or longer life.

Many doctors of fine reputation are doing a disservice to the public. You must exercise, they say. Otherwise you won't be healthy. Get yourself a bike. Run up a half dozen or more flights of stairs a day. Get out and shovel snow. Keep busy on weekends around the house. Paint, garden, walk, do repair work. Don't just sit still. Get going!

Your Formula for Fitness

All you need for fitness is to be within normal weight (which means not overeating); to get into the habit of taking a short nap or two during the day; to get sufficient sleep; take frequent vacations (if only over weekends); get interested in a non-tiring hobby; to leave your brief-case in the office; and to be satisfied with the exertions which come to *you*, and which you do not go out of your way to *seek*, in the course of your day.

I keep telling wives they can keep their husbands alive longer if they don't nag them into taking exercise. Each one finds his own way to relax over the weekend. Some like to work in the garden or play golf or climb mountains. That's all right—if they are physically fit and really enjoy it.

But if your husband prefers to be lazy around the house and do absolutely nothing, that is his way of storing up energy for being the breadwinner during the coming week. Don't suggest that he follow the crowd. Just because John Smith likes to exercise is no reason why your Joe Doakes need to do the same, especially if he abhors physical exertion.

Don't Follow the Crowd

Too many, like sheep, follow the crowd for what's supposed "to be good for you." What's good for *you* is not a secret. You know, without question, what's good and what's bad. Many people think exercise is good for them because it makes them feel so uncomfortable and unhappy. "It must be good," they say. It's identical with the reasoning that "this medicine must be good because it tastes so bad."

People say to me, "Why don't you get out of that rocking chair? People will think you're an old man."

And I say, "Then I've been old for a long time. I've liked rocking chairs (and used them) since I've been a kid."

And so far—knock-knock—I've been as fit and healthy as most of my middle-aged friends who act like boys—and often suffer for it.

I tell them that the "cat can't remain the kitten always."

But I stop right there. Only my lazy friends will really understand what I have been saying. At least I bring them assurance that their way of life is the right one; exposed as they are to continued bombardments in the newspapers, on the radio, television and in magazines that "You'd better exercise or the goblins will get you."

Summary of Chapter

1. Don't resent being called **"Lazy."**
2. Do you engage in sports and exercise only because you are shamed?

3. Overexertion can be deadly for the coronary patient: **Case History.**
4. Human beings come in all shapes, forms—and inclinations.
5. Unfortunately, some people have to learn the hard way.
6. The normal middle-aged heart is not as strong as the normal youngster's.
7. I, too, was not free from exercise-temptation.
8. Remember the injuries suffered by the middle-aged woman and the ski-minded doctor.
9. Middle-aged athletes should be aware of overexertion.
10. Physical exercise and fitness are only necessary for the growing. If you are over 40 you do not have to exercise to promote fitness.
11. Recall the newspaper editor who couldn't sit still.
12. Would you speed at seventy miles per hour on old tires?
13. Consider the sad report of fatalities in the Shriner parade.
14. The 20th-century call to fitness is like an epidemic.
15. We need to be fit only from the neck up.
16. Fitness doesn't prevent serious illness.
17. You get more exercise in your normal day than you realize.
18. You are truly lazy if you are not sensitive to the tag.
19. Many doctors disagree that exercise is necessary for good health.
20. Even Benjamin Franklin was physically lazy.
21. Confessions of a lazy man: **Me.**
22. Review the formula for fitness.

The SECOND Commandment: Thou Shalt Not Be Lazy

Forget it IF:

1. You are over 40 and just hate physical exertion.
2. You have lost your taste for golf, tennis etc.
3. You exercise only because it is supposed to be "good for you."
4. You think it will prevent serious illness.
5. You think it will help cure constipation.
6. You think you will be held up to ridicule.
7. You think it will prevent coronary disease.
8. You think it is evidence you are still a "young feller."
9. You feel like a slacker because of the call for fitness coming out of Washington.

NOTE:

Once and for all, come to

Remember it IF:

1. You are in grade school.
2. You are in high school.
3. You are in college.
4. You have had an accident and need special exercises.
5. You have some deformity which requires special exercises.
6. You have some illness— like arthritis which necessitates exercises.

NOTE:

In spite of what many think, I believe that a good physical foundation is necessary in youngsters. In fact, physical training in the schools is far behind what it should be. Nor should physical development stop in the Freshman year of college. It should be a requirement all through the Senior year.

The SECOND Commandment: Thou Shalt Not Be Lazy (Continued)

terms with yourself. If you really like to move your joints and muscles around, then do so in moderation.

However, if you have been born lazy, or turn lazy in middle-years, then for pity's sakes, be lazy without any remorse. Don't hide your inclination to relax.

After the diploma, what? Any amount of physical exertions up to 30; then a gradual slowing up to 40.

After 40 (whether you are 41 or 80) your own inclination should answer the need for exertion.

3

Thou shalt not
Take Tobacco?

**Check the facts before you give up the
pleasure of smoking.**

The patient reached into his pocket for a pack of cigarettes. He then offered me one. When I accepted he said,
"I really went through the motions of asking you to join
me. Frankly, I didn't think you smoked."

When I asked him why, he said, "After all, you doctors
are in the know. The cause of cancer, heart disease, and
all the rest are as easy as the ABC's to you fellows. With
all the statistics publicized lately relative to the tie-up
between cigarette smoking and heart disease and cancer,
I'm really surprised when any doctor smokes. Of course,
we laymen who like cigarettes have an out. We can just
say we're ignorant about it all—and keep on smoking."

Patients often forget that the doctor is not a completely disassociated animal. He is not one-half doctor and one-half human being. There is no fine line of demarcation. He is all-doctor and all-human-being at one and the same time. Therefore, he has his strong desires and weaknesses—even as you and I.

Personal Feelings

When patients ask me how I feel about tobacco personally, they have a right to the straight-from-the-shoulder reply. Many of them believe: "What's good enough for the doctor—healthwise—is good enough for me." I tell them that's poor reasoning. Nevertheless, here goes. Here are my own reactions to the tobacco question.

I have been a steady smoker since the age of 18. Every few years I would test my will to see whether I was man or mouse. I would forego tobacco for three or four weeks or months. Perhaps I could blame a guilty conscience. After telling so many sick people who needed to stop smoking to stop, I felt that I should, in all fairness, give up the weed in penance. But only temporarily! Then, the trial period over, I would begin to smoke again.

In college I must have been quite a pipe smoker. Whenever I put away my pipe for a few hours, friends would say, "What's the matter? Where's the good old pipe?" As I came into medical practice, there was less time for the pipe during the day. I switched to cigarettes—with an occasional pipeful at night.

One Christmas, quite a few years ago, a number of patients who grow tobacco kindly deluged me with gifts of cigars. I soon grew to enjoy their taste.

At this point you may say, "That's all right, but remember that was years before the appalling statistics on cancer and heart disease. How do you feel about smoking now? Are you still a heavy smoker?"

The answer is that I was *never* a heavy smoker—and am not now. For years my daily quota has been about ten cigarettes a day, with an occasional pipeful at night. On the days I smoke three or four cigars I never smoke a pipe, and take perhaps two or three cigarettes.

Why haven't I, as a doctor, stopped smoking? The reason must be evident: I am not convinced in my own mind that the direct relationship between smoking and cancer has been proved. At the exact moment that incontrovertible proof comes I shall be among the first to throw my pipes, cigars and cigarettes into the waste basket—forever. Following which I shall at high noon shout the news from some building at the busiest corner of town: "Tobacco is dangerous to health and life beyond a doubt."

But as that moment is not yet here I shall continue, in moderation, to enjoy the pleasure of smoking so highly praised by Barrie.

What I Tell Patients

In effect, here is what I tell patients. You are a fool to smoke if you have sinus trouble, chronic bronchitis, emphysema, asthma, hypertension, Buerger's disease (a disease of the arteries in the extremities), stomach ulcer or coronary disease. Yet I do not point a finger menacingly and say, "You *must* do this; you *mustn't* do that." I think we doctors can only *suggest* the best way of life for each individual. We have no right to live their lives for them.

The wonderful Sir Winston Churchill, in his late 80's sustained a broken thigh-bone from a fall out of bed. Doctors had advised that he forego his customary cigar and brandy. I said to a colleague, "That will kill him faster than any complications the fracture can bring." Fortunately, within hours, common sense took over at the bedside. A newspaper article described that he was again enjoying his customary brandy and cigar.

However, I do tell the two- or three-pack-a-day smoker this: "If I smoked over two packs a day and a doctor asked me to cut down to one, I'd certainly try. And if I couldn't limit myself, I don't think I'd deserve to smoke at all. I'd quit."

Coming from a physician, what I am saying may sound like heresy. Nevertheless, it isn't. I have never advocated smoking. I have always outlined its potential dangers so people could make their choice. But at this stage of our investigations, I do not think it fair to take away a pleasure from Mr. A. just because it may prove harmful to Mr. B. As there is no test which will show where the danger lies, it is the right of the human being involved to make the choice, and not of his doctor.

Perhaps the most usual question asked us doctors these days is this: "Is smoking really harmful? Do you think I had better quit?" The answer, of course, depends upon the identity of the questioner. Smoking, I have been trying to say, is neither all good nor all bad. For example, let me give you some specific answers to some patients.

Some Specific Answers

Many young women who are pregnant wonder if smoking will harm the child. I know of no evidence that implicates tobacco here except a recent study which shows that it may influence the weight of the child.

Dr. C. R. Lowe, in the *British Medical Journal,* wrote that he had obtained the smoking histories from 2,042 pregnant mothers who were delivered in Birmingham maternity hospitals. It was found that the mean weight of infants of mothers who smoked regularly throughout pregnancy was six ounces less than that of infants of mothers who never smoked during pregnancy. Therefore, it doesn't seem that moderate smoking will in any way jeopardize the pregnancy—or the child.

A man with chronic catarrh, sinusitis and morning cough wonders if he should stop smoking. The answer is evident. I tell him that he really doesn't need a doctor's reply to that question. What he is looking for is an excuse to continue a habit that is unquestionably detrimental to his health and comfort. If you have ever been a heavy smoker with similar symptoms you know how much better you feel when you give up the weed. Nevertheless, many of these people say, "I guess I'd be more comfortable if I quit, but I enjoy it so much I'd rather smoke and put up with catarrh and morning cough."

I recall a man with chronic bronchitis and asthma who was the most miserably uncomfortable man you would want to see. Yet, he continued to smoke, saying, "I know cigarettes will be the death of me, but I just can't stop."

When an apparently healthy individual asks me if he should continue or stop, I tell him to measure his pleasure in smoking and compare it with his discomforts—if any. The choice is his. We doctors don't have the right to set ourselves up as moralists and order a blanket embargo on all smoking. We should, I believe, continue to lay all the cards face up. But the final decision in a healthy person (and in a sick one) is his alone to make.

Most People Aware of Dangers

Most persons are now aware of the potential dangers of smoking. Papers, books, magazines and other media have stressed the apparent relationship between smoking and cancer and heart disease. Many medical men fully believe that the man who smokes cigarettes is inviting cancer of the lungs or an attack of coronary thrombosis. Others will not agree to this unless they have better proof than "apparent" proof as indicated by statistics. They do not feel morally justified in taking away man's pleasures without definitely convincing evidence.

According to a note in the *AMA News,* a national survey by the American Cancer Society shows that only forty-three percent of physicians smoke cigarettes regularly and five percent occasionally. Of the twenty-nine percent who used to smoke, a large majority have quit during the last nine years. Thirty-three percent of the MD's said that cigarette smoking "definitely" was a major cause of lung cancer, thirty-one percent said "probably."

I belong to this latter group. When a healthy man asks me about smoking, I tell him about the potential dangers and leave the choice to him. I do not say: **Thou Shalt Not Take Tobacco.**

Dangerous for Buerger's Disease

However, if there is a definite contra-indication, as coronary disease or thromboangitis obliterans (Buerger's

—commonly called "leg-artery disease") I can be as tough in such cases as apparently lax in dealing with healthy persons. If you came to me with Buerger's I'd say you have no choice. I will make it for you. Stop! Quit! Desist! If you continue to smoke you will never get well.

I'd tell you about one man with Buerger's who already had one leg amputated. Nevertheless, he continued to smoke against advice. I saw him about two years later with both legs off. He was wheeling himself along in a chair, a cigarette hanging from his lips. He had made his choice. Depending upon how well you are, you will have to make yours: to smoke or not to smoke. But sometimes there is only one sensible answer: Stop!

I admit that the practice of smoking may be filthy and obnoxious to non-smokers. But so is excessive horn-tootin' obnoxious to many of us; so is boorishness; and loud-mouthness; and any form of selfishness and inconsiderateness of our neighbors or strangers.

Yet, living in the world as it is, we must learn to put up with these deficiencies in our fellow human beings. Else, we would be in a constant tug of war with each other; every other person trying to transform us into "acceptable persons."

I Do Not Take Sides

Coming back to the question of tobacco, I can foresee no law on the horizon which will prohibit the use of tobacco. It would be a greater failure than Prohibition of an earlier year. Meanwhile, it is the duty of the capable and honest physician to present the problem to the public impartially.

It is true that the incidence of heart disease and cancer of the lung has progressed rapidly; that it has kept step with cigarette sales. But it is also true that there are more cars spewing out carbon monoxide fumes and other gases on our city streets. I feel more uncomfortable and anxious sitting in my car behind a large bus in traffic, than I do when I light up a smoke.

The consumption of vitamins has increased. Shall we blame heart and lung diseases on that? Men are using electric shavers in greater numbers to parallel the increase of heart and lung disease. Shall we point the finger to breathing in the hair-dust while shaving. We could say the reason why men get more lung cancer than women is because we shave and they don't.

As I have said, many good doctors have given up smoking, and advise their patients to do so, because they are convinced that tobacco is harmful. I agree that it may be harmful—but who is to say which healthy person it harms? Just as many excellent physicians take the stand, "They haven't proved it to me yet." So they go on smoking.

Not Preaching Dangerous Doctrine

What I am writing here will distress a great number of people. Laymen who have been frightened into giving up tobacco will feel that I am preaching a dangerous doctrine. Some members of the medical profession may think I am undoing the good that has been done in warning the populace against smoking. Nevertheless, I believe it is only fair to give you both sides of the argument.

Life is relatively short. It is not only foolhardy, but

wasteful of our pleasures, to forswear them on flimsy evidence. I do not go about preaching that non-smokers should begin to smoke. In fact, I tell them they might be better off without the habit. But I do try to bring a modicum of comfort to those who really enjoy a smoke— but find that fear and a guilty conscience are taking all the fun out of smoking.

Mrs. L. says, "I have a friend who has high blood pressure and limits herself to no more than four cigarettes a day. She has never gone over this quota for years. If you were her doctor, would you ask her to stop? She enjoys them so much, especially, after eating."

I told her that I would not ask her to stop. You can't practice medicine "by the book." Common sense is vitally important. In this instance why take a simple pleasure (only four cigarettes daily) away from a patient who has sufficient will power not to go overboard in her smoking. That's almost like punishing a child for being good!

The Chain Smoker

Mrs. M. says: "My sister, a widow who lives with me, is a chain smoker. Never have I seen anyone smoke a cigarette like she does. She lights it and keeps it in her mouth until ready to dispose of the butt. I have asked her why she smokes this way. She says that once she laid a cigarette down and almost burned up her place. Since then she says she has been 'playing safe.' She always complains about her throat bothering her and lately she has been hoarse. I must confess she is getting on my nerves. Have you any suggestions on handling her?"

I warned her that persistent hoarseness and pain in the

throat may be evidence of beginning serious trouble. I spelled it out for her: **cancer.** Tell your sister that, I said. Not only should she stop acting like a smoke-stack; it's time that she let a throat specialist take a good look. And perhaps a good diagnostician. Having the house burn down is not as catastrophic as developing incurable disease of the throat or lungs.

In my experience, chain smokers are usually tense persons. It's their way of letting off steam. In a roundabout way, treating her nervousnses may relieve and neutralize her intense desire to smoke all the time.

Another patient says: "I keep reading that cigarettes are the real culprits where cancer of the lungs is concerned. I happen to smoke a pipe. Does that relieve me of all fear that my personal tobacco habit may get me into some trouble?"

Less Danger in Pipe and Cigars?

I tell him that whether the reason is that there's something bad in the cigarette paper or cigarette tobacco itself; or that cigarette smokers tend to inhale more deeply: the fact remains that, according to statistics, at least, cigarettes and the inhalation of noxious gases which surround us in our modern civilization are the villans where cancer of the lungs is concerned.

But your pipe habit has some inherent dangers, too. We believe that the constant irritation of the hot pipe-stem may be in some way tied in with cancer of the lips. Cigar smokers are more liable to get cancer of the tongue. Do you chew snuff or tobacco? There's greater likelihood of cancer of the inside of the cheeks.

In a paper given at a meeting of the American Heart Association the speaker stressed that the potential dangers of cigarette smoking was greater than for pipe and cigar smokers.

I wish I could say that cigar or pipe smoking are innocuous habits and that you can smoke these to your heart's content. But I can't. I really don't understand why cigarettes are supposed to be so harmful and continually get a good, stiff sentence of scientific disapproval, while pipes and cigars go scot free with a pat on the back and a judgment of "not guilty."

Until we have the true answer about all forms of tobacco, I am not going overboard in my advice to patients. I won't say "better switch from cigarettes to pipe or cigar." Whatever your present smoking habit, I will say that you will be better off if you smoke moderately than if you overdo it. Perhaps the best advice, if you are already ill, is to quit. As the woman said, whose guest burned a hole in her new davenport with a cigarette, "Smoking's a nasty habit." Although I smoke moderately, if it were my davenport I'd agree.

Tobacco and Coronary Disease

Mrs. K. says: "What do you think of tobacco in a patient who has recently recovered from an attack of coronary thrombosis? Is it dangerous? Will it predispose to another attack?" These questions arise in the minds of most coronary patients who are smokers.

"My husband has me worried. He is stubborn. He will not give up his cigarettes. He smokes at least a pack and a half a day."

When I was just beginning practice I treated a business man who recovered nicely from his coronary thrombosis. Previous to his attack he smoked at least two packs a day. In a long bedside talk I explained that tobacco was taboo from now on. He agreed to stop.

I recall that he met me at the door a few days later when I was making a house call. He was smoking a cigarette. I asked him how many he had had that day. "About a pack," he said, as unconcernedly as if he had never heard my advice.

Being young and perhaps overly conscientious, I told him that I would not continue to treat him. I suggested he get another doctor. He did. The fact that he died about six months later did not prove that the cigarettes were his coffin nails. But I have always been certain that tobacco "never did coronary patients any good."

Since my experience with this patient, I have learned that doctors can't (or at least, shouldn't) *make* patients do as they advise. All we can do is give you what we hope is good advice and trust that you will follow it. Now that I am more mellow, I warn you against smoking if you have coronary disease. But I tell you that the choice is yours. I don't lay down the law: "Don't smoke or else!"

In reference to tobacco, I have been reading some notes which appeared in the *Journal of the American Geriatric Society:*

"U.S. statistical studies indicate that while a 13.5 percent increase in the incidence of lung cancer has been noted among heavy smokers, a 52 percent increase in deaths from coronary artery diseases has been chalked up by the same group.

"Similar studies in Great Britain show a 12.7 percent increase in lung cancer, 39.4 percent increase in coronary artery disease, 17 percent increase in other circulatory diseases among heavy smokers."

In commenting on such data, a few years ago, Dr. Irving S. Wright, Professor of Clinical Medicine at Cornell University Medical College wrote:

"The medical profession should look harder at these data. Those concerned with cancer have been looking at the lung cancer aspect, but have cardiologists been looking at the deaths from coronary disease with the same intensive interest? I believe they have not."

However, now they are looking harder. In the United States many studies seem to point the accusing finger at cigarettes as having a bad effect on the heart and arteries. The Royal College of Physicians in England issued a report in 1962 that says in part: "It seems reasonable at present to agree with the recent statement of the committee on smoking and cardiovascular disease of the American Heart Association, that present evidence 'strongly suggests that heavy cigarette smoking may contribute to or accelerate the development of coronary disease or its complications,' at least in men under the age of 55."

If you are at all concerned about the ill effects of tobacco, in the present state of our knowledge, I'd say better look more to your heart and arteries than to fear of lung cancer. I am not at all convinced that tobacco is the important factor in lung cancer rather than air pollution.

Choose Your Poison

Granted that the tobacco plant contains the following: pyridine, formic acid, malic acid, oxalic acid, citric acid, fumaric acid, succinic acid, acetic acid, quinnic acid, caffeic acid, nitric acid, formaldehyde, methyl alcohol, arsenic, acetone, phenols, ammonia, carbon monoxide, tars, nicotine and additional substances: which are enough to frighten any imaginative fellow and cause him to quickly dispose of his smoking paraphernalia.

But I ask myself why doctors haven't been seeing more cancer of the tongue, mouth and lip? Why should tobacco irritants spare these?

Consider air pollution. As I said earlier, when I get tied up in traffic behind a large bus or other cars emitting gaseous fumes, I say to myself that every day, in the large cities of the U.S., thousands of innocent citizens are being exposed to irritants and poisons of which they are not aware.

For example, consider Los Angeles. According to a report put out by the magazine *Patterns of Disease,* here is what happens in one day in Los Angeles, when the exhausts of autos have got in their dirty work. In 24 hours they emit 965 tons of hydrocarbons, 250 tons of nitrogen oxides, 19 tons of sulfur dioxide, 6,850 tons of carbon monoxide and 27 tons of aerosols. It is not necessary to explain the effects of each contaminant, except to say that taken together they most certainly must have something to do with bronchitis, lung cancer and other respiratory ailments. I am happy that at last, scientists are working to discover some way to neutralize most of these air pollutants. The solution can't come too fast.

According to Dr. Geoffrey Dean of Port Elizabeth, South Africa, cigarette smoking and polluted air interact to produce lung cancer. He noted that South Africa has clean air, and British cities are dirty and filled with smog. When smokers moved from Britain to South Africa they had twice the death rate of South Africans who smoked as many cigarettes.

And in an article of the *Journal of the American Medical Association* (May 5, 1962) by Drs. Seymour M. Farber and Roger H. L. Wilson of San Francisco, called "Air Contamination, a Respiratory Hazard," they say:

> "Although a connection between air pollution and non-malignant respiratory diseases can only be proposed tentatively, the connection between air pollution and cancer of the respiratory system is as sure as statistical studies can make it. Studies from all parts of the world converge up on one conclusion, that air pollution plays a substantial role in the etiology of bronchogenic carcinoma (lung cancer)."

This perhaps explains why there is more lung cancer in the cities than in the small towns.

Tired of Statistics?

Statistics! Statistics! By now you must be tired of them —whether they seem to support you or go against your feeling about tobacco. I'm fed up with them myself because I've been reading more reports than you have. But I wanted you to see both sides.

(I am writing this at 10 P.M. I have just lit a cigarette and am taking inventory—for the purpose in hand—of my tobacco consumption during the day. I have smoked three cigars and this is my fifth cigarette. I realize I am in the position of the braggart and poseur who stands out in a field during a lightning storm and dares God to strike him dead. But I do not tell you this in such spirit. My obituary notices may prove me wrong—but I smoke without fear and without being conscience-stricken. But that gaseous traffic I was in today—that scares me!)

Many Things Don't Add Up

Many questions raise so many doubts about just how dangerous tobacco is for the human being. For example, why haven't leading insurance companies raised life insurance rates on smokers? In fact, why do they issue policies to smokers at all? Why is cancer of the lip rarely found in the Tyrol where men smoke clay pipes continuously? Why, in one study conducted in Britain, was less lung cancer found in cigarette smokers who habitually inhaled than in those who didn't?

I recall a statement made by Dr. Maude Slye, famous investigator, who concluded: "Not only is there hereditary susceptibility to cancer, but there is also hereditary unsusceptibility. Thus thousands are by heredity free from the tendency to cancer."

I asked myself these questions: "Is a man placid because he smokes a pipe, or does he prefer a pipe because his is a quiet, unruffled disposition?

Does tobacco cause heart disease, or is it the stressful individual who reaches for cigarette after cigarette himself the real cause? Does Mr. A. get cancer because he is the susceptible one—and for that reason alone?

Highway Tragedies

Cancer takes about 270,000 lives annually in the United States. Lung cancer struck down about 45,000 Americans in 1961. I needn't remind you about the beginning commotion in Washington that we had better do something about it. I've heard talk about actually banning tobacco—a kind of Prohibition all over again. We tend to get hysterical about one danger and completely ignore a more certain one.

For example, for years I have been distressed at the wanton killings on the highways of the innocent by the automobile. There is no question at all there. We have no doubts—as in lung cancer. Yet, what steps has the government taken to actually prevent the needless deaths and disfigurations? They cause more tragedies than does cancer of the lung. The cold war in traffic has been a hot war since the turn of the century and—until lately, at least—we have sat by complacently until tragedy struck in our own home.

I think of something else. Years ago doctors thought that cigarette smoking caused tuberculosis. What has happened to that theory? Another thing: the consumption of cigarettes has gone up at least a thousand per cent in the past few decades but the percentage of lip cancer in women has remained about the same as when they didn't smoke.

Vernon A. Butcher made this interesting observation: "If one visits the tobacco farms of the U.S. or the West

Indies, he will frequently find that the oldest Negro on the plantation is the greatest smoker. If, as some statisticians claim, the use of tobacco shortens the span of life, how can we account for the longevity of many heavy smokers unless we assume that tobacco is a poison of peculiar whims, shortening the lives of some men but having little or no effect on others?" (*Un*susceptibility—remember?)

Tobacco Lovers—Tobacco Haters

Tobacco was discovered by Columbus in 1492 when he observed the use of this plant by the Indians. Spain, Portugal and Italy were the first European countries to sample this Indian weed. England and France soon followed.

But there were the dissenters in those days, too. Consider the famous denunciation of tobacco by James I of England, called *Counterblaste of Tobacco:*

"There cannot be a more base, and yet hurtful corruption in a country than this barbarous and beastly habit borrowed from wild Indians, a habit unnatural, urgent, expensive, unclean, loathsome to the eye, hateful to the nose, harmful to the brain, dangerous to the lungs—and in the black, stinking fume thereof nearest resembling the horrible Stygian smoke of the pit that is bottomless."

(Perhaps you have seen many of his counterparts today.)

As one aptly expressed it: "A matter of conjecture and prejudice"—by those who hate tobacco.

But there have been tobacco lovers down through the ages, too. And these lovers seemed to court the pipe or cigar, rather than the cigarette—which they didn't seem to hold in high esteem.

Mark Twain smoked about 300 cigars a month and when he was 70 declared, "I have made it a rule never to smoke more than one cigar at a time."

General Grant smoked about 25 cigars a day. Lincoln telegraphed him August 17, 1864, before an important battle, "Hold on with bulldog grip, and chew and smoke as much as possible." After Lee's surrender, from all over America came gifts totalling about 30,000 cigars.

Izaak Walton, a heavy smoker, died at 90. Hobbes, famous philosopher, smoked 12 pipes a day but lived to be 92. Carlyle was an inveterate smoker and died at 86. And how about Churchill and his cigar? And Bertrand Russell and his pipe?

Thomas Huxley said, "There is no more harm in a pipe than there is in a cup of tea. You may poison yourself by drinking too much green tea, and kill yourself by eating too many beefsteaks."

For many, the cigar or pipe is one of the creature comforts of existence—a kind companion and a solace. Bulwer Lytton said that, "A cigar is as great a comfort to a man as a good cry to a woman."

Guizot, the French historian was sitting in his study one day smoking a pipe. A lady called on him, and finding him smoking, exclaimed, "What! You smoke and yet have arrived at so great an age?"

"Ah, madame," replied Guizot, "if I had not smoked I should have been dead ten years ago."

Man Is Jealous of His Pleasures

Then as now there were the pros and the cons. People took sides in heat, as they often do today. If you will examine it, you will find that most of men's pleasures have been clawed at some time or other by those who could not live and let live. Children learn it early when their comic books are forbidden; men learn it when their books are banned in Boston. To many, sex is degrading; alcohol a poison; TV a national disgrace; dancing, a return to the primitive; tranquilizers nothing but dope; and the movies and the theater disgraceful.

But man is jealous of his pleasures. It is his way of self-preservation. When sex disappears, we will. So will we if books disappear; if the dance and the theater founder.

Continued existence may not depend upon tobacco but I have a hunch that Sir Walter Raleigh was correct in his prediction when he lit his pipe and said, "We are today lighting a candle which by God's blessing will never be put out."

I spoke to an interesting gentleman who sat contentedly smoking his pipe on a park bench. I happened to be smoking my pipe at the time so there was an instant communion of good spirit and no need for formal introduction.

After saying that cigarettes are harmful because smokers invariably inhale, he said pipe smokers and cigar fanciers rarely do—and therefore don't get into any trouble. He continued: "I am seventy-four years of age and have smoked for about sixty years. When first starting, my

mother pleaded with me never to smoke cigarettes, because they were in those days known as 'coffin nails.'
I promised and have religiously kept this promise in her
memory. In my case the smoking of a pipe or cigar acts
as a tranquilizer and I believe an aid to digestion. Does
this make sense?"

Does it? Only time will tell.

The sick man who continues to smoke may be a fool.
So may be the healthy man who forsakes the joy of
smoking because flimsy evidence influences him to quit
without reason.

Listen to columnist Jack Kofoed of the *Miami Herald:*

"They found that cigarette smoking is blamed for
mouth and lung cancer; milk, ice cream and cheese for
cholesterol and heart disease. Now in Iceland it is as-
serted that the only people who get cancer of the stomach
are those who eat too much smoked salmon and trout.

"It's getting so that if there's anything you enjoy, like
smoking, or having a Bloody Mary before dinner, or eating stuff you like, experts will warn that indulgence is
bound to take years off your life. So, why worry about a
few extra years, when other experts devise bombs to end
life in the blink of an eye? Eat, drink and be merry, without a twitch about nicotine or cholesterol, for tomorrow it
may be the hydrogen bomb."

Summary of Chapter

1. The doctor who smokes does so because he is one-
   half doctor and one-half human being.
2. I have been a moderate smoker since age 18.
3. I tell patients they are fools to smoke if they have
   Buerger's disease, sinus trouble, chronic bronchitis,

emphysema, asthma, stomach ulcer, high blood pressure, coronary disease.

4. Anyone who can't cut down to less than one pack a day should not smoke at all.

5. Smoking produces no great harm to mother or child.

6. If you are healthy, the choice (to smoke or not) is up to you alone.

7. Most people are aware of potential dangers to the lungs, heart and arteries. They make their choice with eyes open.

8. The chain smoker is asking for trouble: major or minor.

9. Pipes and cigars seem less dangerous than cigarettes.

10. Cigarettes certainly don't help coronary disease. Cause it? That's another story.

11. Not only cigarette smoke, but city air cause foul pollution.

12. Statistics? Many things don't add up.

13. We are excited about lung cancer yet take needless highway tragedies as a matter of course.

14. There always have been—and always will be—tobacco haters and tobacco lovers.

15. Man is jealous of his pleasures.

The THIRD Commandment: Thou Shalt Not Take Tobacco

Forget it IF:

1. You have had a recent physical and your doctor finds no definite contra-indication.
2. If you really enjoy tobac-co.
3. You limit your smoking to pipe or cigar.
4. You do not inhale when you smoke cigarettes.
5. You can limit yourself to less than 10 cigarettes a day.
6. You have read all the pros and cons and have come to a decision in the face of all the threats to health—proved and un-proved.
7. If you have no morning cough or other discom-forts you can directly trace to smoking.

Remember it IF:

1. If you are actually fright-ened by all you have been reading and hear-ing.
2. If you don't actually en-joy tobacco.
3. If your doctor has asked you to stop smoking for any of the following specific reasons: a) sinus trouble b) bronchitis c) emphysema d) asthma e) ulcer f) coronary throm-bosis g) angina pectoris h) high blood pressure i) evidence of severe throat irritation or other irrita-tion.
4. If you—or others around you—are allergic to to-bacco.
5. If—and there are no ifs, ands and buts here—you have Buerger's disease.

The THIRD Commandment: Thou Shalt Not Take Tobacco (Continued)

NOTE:

For some tobacco smoking (or chewing or sniffing) is a filthy habit. For others, it is one of life's great pleasures. To smoke or not to smoke? Only the patient himself can answer the question—after the doctor has laid before him all the evidence which relates to him.

NOTE:

Many persons who have been told not to smoke because of specific contra-indications continue to do so at their own risk. For example, the patient with Buerger's disease actually goes about killing himself with tobacco.

4

Thou shalt not
Take Alcohol?

In many cases, alcohol is the best medicine.

Whenever he has occasion to introduce me to one of his friends, Mr. A., who is 84, says mischievously, "When I was a young man of 60, my doctor here made me take up a bad habit: drinking. I remember I was complaining of insomnia at the time. Nothing seemed to help. Pills always gave me an awful hangover the next day. He told me to try a small glass of sherry or port to wash down one aspirin tablet. It was so wonderful that I've taken this advice every night of my life since then, and I've slept like a baby."

When the effect of his little story sinks in he adds, looking around at me semi-seriously, "But I keep wondering how this treatment will affect me later in life. I mean, will I become a chronic alcoholic?"

12-Year-Old Drinks Beer

And when I think of Mr. A. I recall Mrs. G., who was in with her 12-year-old son. It is a case history at the other end of the spectrum. Concerned about her boy, she said, "What is your opinion about children being allowed to drink alcoholic beverages? My husband has been permitting our Jimmy to drink a bottle of beer with his dinner. Don't you think this is entirely too much alcohol for a youngster who weighs only 90 pounds? I can't reason with my husband. He claims that if a child drinks at home with his meals he will never think of drinking as a novelty when he grows older. What do you think about it?"

I told her that it actually gives me the creeps whenever I see a number of boys at a high school party standing around with beer bottles in hand while their parents calmly pass the sandwiches—apparently unaware of the spectre of chronic alcoholism which is surreptitiously planting seeds in some of these kids.

As for her 12-year-old, you can imagine what I had to say to her husband when I called him later. Fortunately, being an old patient, he listened and didn't cut me off. He said he'd take the daily portion of beer away from his son.

When I saw Jimmy weeks later he told me confidentially, "I'm glad you told Pop to stop giving me the stuff. I hated it at first, but was just beginning to like it. Now that I know it's a bad habit, I promise not to drink until I'm an old man."

Alcohol a Boon or a Poison

For over 25 years in practice, I have treated alcohol as a drug with the respect it deserves. It can be both a poison and a boon to mankind. Those who begin drinking when young court the well-known disaster of chronic alcoholism; those who do not drink until middle-age may find actual medicinal value from its use.

In all the years I have been prescribing moderate intake of alcohol in those past 40, I do not recall one patient whom I have converted into a chronic alcoholic. One psychiatrist friend told me he had never seen chronic alcoholism as a problem in anyone past 45 who had never been an alcoholic before 45. He said, "I've just reviewed 500 of my cases in the alcoholism clinic. Only two in the entire series said they did not begin to drink until after 40. But on further questioning these two admitted they had been heavy drinkers since their twenties."

Many Can't Take It

Why do I prescribe alcohol after 45 in most patients? (Of course, there are exceptions: those with extreme high blood pressure; ulcer patients; gall bladder patients; gout sufferers; chauffeurs and others who drive a car often; those with kidney or liver disease; and especially those who are emotionally unstable.) I prescribe it because I think it is one of the safest and best drugs to cut the rope of tension—and when you prevent tension you reduce the possibilities of coronary thrombosis, anginal attacks, stroke, hypertension, diabetes, hyperthyroidism.

Patients I have treated for years—having brought them through attacks of severe illness like pneumonia or heart disease—have told me: "Do you know the best advice you ever gave me? Do you know what I've appreciated more than anything else? When you told me years ago to take a highball before dinner."

And I know exactly what they mean. I expressed it this way a few years ago, which indicates, I believe, that I see both sides of the problem:

Alcohol Can Cause Grief

Doctors find themselves on the spot when they prescribe liquor. Few know better than they do how much grief can be caused by excessive drinking. They see the bewildered, frightened children; they know of the lost jobs and insolvent businesses; they try to cheer the sober partner as the other unconsciously tears down the pillars of marriage; they stand by and observe the frustration, helplessness and loss of hope—and finally, illness and death.

In the United States there are about 50 million social drinkers; three million or more excessive drinkers; and at least 750,000 who suffer from chronic alcoholism.

Yet, we doctors know there is another side to it. We recognize that alcohol can also do much good. It is an important part of the doctor's therapeutic armamentarium.

To begin with, we must remember that every drug the doctor prescribes has potentialities for harm. The layman knows that too many morphine, phenobarbital, bromide, aspirin or thyroid pills can be harmful, too. That even an apparently harmless concoction like bicarbonate of soda water is known to be life-shortening, if taken often enough, for some heart and high blood pressure sufferers.

Helpful Too

Likewise, alcohol is a two-edged sword: one dull, the other sharp. Before accepting or rejecting it, there are a few things you should know. In moderate amounts liquor is an appetizer and stomachic. A martini "makes" many a dinner a social function. For the elderly, alcohol seems to provide a new lease on life.

It produces a sense of well-being. Where there was taciturnity before there is loquaciousness; where there was the masklike, expressionless face, there is now the smile. For a time, the elder becomes again the gay blade and "business-producer" of yesteryear. Alcohol is often invaluable in translating discomfort into comfort when anginal pains grip the chest.

But I find that alcohol's chief value is in fighting tension. I have found that there are few better ways of cutting the strong, thick rope of tension that ties people to their work than by taking an ounce of sherry, a glass of ale or beer, or a shot of scotch or bourbon before dinner. It eases away cares and fatigue, stimulates appetite, makes food taste better, enlivens conversation, brightens the outlook.

I repeat, over the years hundreds upon hundreds of patients have told me, in all sobriety, how much the daily ounce or two of liquor has added to the fullness and enjoyment of their lives.

I do not question my own experience with patients, but it is always reassuring to know one is not alone in his experience.

Therefore, I have been especially interested in what a symposium of noted sociologists and biochemists speaking at the University of California School of Medicine found.

Dr. William Dock of New York said: "I have felt that what is needed in retreats for ailing or aged people, and even in city hospitals, is a regular alcohol ration." (On my medical services in the wards of the McCook Memorial and the Mt. Sinai hospitals of Hartford, Conn. I recall many elderly patients apparently dying of pneumonia— in the days before sulfa drugs and antibiotics—who were given the courage to continue fighting because of the euphoria produced by a tablespoonful of alcohol which I prescribed to be taken every three or four hours.)

And at the same symposium the noted Yale physiologist, Leon A. Greenberg said: "Alcohol is the safest, most available tranquilizer we have." (Often, in a choice between prescribing tranquilizers in pill form and whiskey in small doses, my experience has been that alcohol has worked better.)

Acts as Tranquilizer

I recall an industrialist who had got into the habit of popping tranquilizers into his mouth about 4 P.M. every day. He said, "That's about the time that the pressures mount up. Not only am I about all-in on the job, but I have to face a lot of tension when I get home. So I have learned to fortify myself with some tranquilizers. If I take them about four, they begin to ease me up before I leave here around six, and things are smoother at home. I also take two sleeping pills every night, although I hate to, because I feel drugged through half of the morning."

He impressed me as the type who would soon be doubling his doses of tranquilizers, and probably taking three and four sleeping pills at night.

As he was 48, and had never had alcohol before on "moral" grounds, I suggested that he give up the tranquilizers and take some liquor instead. I suggested to his wife that she meet him at the door with a highball containing an ounce of scotch or bourbon; that she hold off dinner until he had had time to sit back with the evening paper for a half hour; that she join him with a glass of sherry herself. Also, I prescribed some sherry before he retired.

That was years ago. Neither he nor his wife have increased their daily intake of alcohol. He, like our 84-year-old friend, has slept like a baby. Evening tensions at home have disappeared. He has not had to take tranquilizers.

Alcoholism an Old Problem

Alcoholism is not a recent problem. There is reference to drunkenness in the ninth chapter of Genesis. (Of Noah: "And he drank of the wine, and was drunken.") And the use of alcohol as a medicine goes back far into the Dark Ages. Before anesthetics, alcohol was used as a narcotic to help patients withstand painful operations.

Some say that the origin of alcohol goes back 200 million years to the Paleozoic era. By that time the necessary materials for its formation appeared on earth: water, plant sugars and yeast. As we all know now, it is the yeast which sets in motion the fermentation of various vegetable sugars (berries, honey, grain, fruit, etc.) to produce alcohol. According to Ernest Crawley, English sociologist, "The use of corn (grain) for the preparation of fermented liquor is perhaps almost as early as its use for food." And Professor Edgar Andersen at Washington University in St. Louis has said, "Man may well have been a brewer before he was a baker."

The Greek historian Herodotus writing about the Egyptian banqueting customs about 500 years before the birth of Christ says: "After dinner a man carries round an image of a corpse in a coffin, painted and carved in exact imitation, a cubit or two cubits long. This he shows to each of the company, saying: 'Drink and make merry, but look on this; for such shalt thou be when thou art dead.' "

Writing even earlier, a Chinese philosopher said of alcohol: "Men will not do without it. To prohibit it and secure total abstinence from it is beyond the power even of sages. Here, therefore, we have warnings on the abuse of it." (And the warnings recommended moderation.)

People Take Sides

For centuries—long before Prohibition in the United States—men took sides, heatedly, on the good and bad effects of alcohol. To this day there are many who vehemently defend or attack alcohol, neither on scientific or moral grounds, but on preconceived notions which close ears and eyes against contrary opinions.

For example, Lord D'Abernon in his book *Alcohol: Its*

Action on the Human Organism wrote: "Alcohol is an ungrateful subject. Most people who are interested in the subject are already partisans on the one side or the other, and no body of impartial opinion exists which is ready to be guided by scientific inquiry. The majority of those who would give any attention to original work on the subject would do so less to gain knowledge than to find arms and argument to support their preconceived opinion."

And Raymond G. McCarthy and Edgar M. Douglass support this view in their *Alcohol and Social Responsibility* when they write: "The distorted ideas about alcohol which are commonly held among the public in general are largely founded on emotionalism."

It is for these reasons that it is often difficult to convince people who need alcohol as a medicine to take it. They refuse on "moral grounds." They know that alcohol is of the Devil himself so they won't take it.

Good for Angina

I recall a man in his early fifties who was taking over two dozen nitroglycerine tablets every day for angina pectoris. As I have found alcohol to be of help in many such patients I recommended that he take an ounce of liquor three times a day. He refused. He told me he was afraid of becoming an alcoholic like his father was. I told him there was little chance of this happening. That the control of his angina was more important at this time than vague fears of the future.

He was stubborn and afraid. When I showed him a statement by Dr. Paul D. White who was much in the news at the time as the physician of President Eisenhower, he at last agreed. Dr. White had written: "An ounce or two of whiskey, brandy or rum may give rapid relief from angina pectoris, usually in the course of a very few minutes."

We know that tension is an important consideration in attacks of angina. After taking the liquor as recommended, our patient got along on less than a half dozen nitroglycerine tablets a day.

If you can limit yourself to no more than an ounce or two a day, alcohol will contribute to good living. Many people are fearful that even moderate amounts will cause cirrhosis of the liver. There is no adequate scientific proof that this is so. Many years ago Dr. Raymond Pearl of Johns Hopkins indicated that moderate drinkers live longer than abstainers. I believe that modern statistical studies would show that alcohol has often done much to prevent such serious diseases as coronary artery disease and hypertensive disease that are due to excess tension and stress.

Welcome Medicine for Elderly

In the aging, especially, have I seen its good effects. Too many old people mope along from day to day without any enthusiasms, without appetite, without any joy in living whatever. A tablespoonful of whiskey three or four times a day is often the difference between just existing and living in these people.

Listen to experts H. W. Haggard and E. M. Jellinek of Yale. These doctors wrote: "When older people use alcohol in suitable moderation and low concentrations it increases their desire for food. There is mild euphoria (well-being), a cheerfulness, and decrease of anxiety; the feeling of chilliness is lessened by the flow of blood to the skin, and the mild sedative action of the alcohol relieves some of the aches and pains."

I remember a man of 65 who sustained a coronary thrombosis. He became depressed and, according to his family "not fit to live with." He was anxious, non-talkative, and completely non-social. Neither sedatives nor tranquilizers did any good. He lived and acted like a dried-up vegetable.

When I was called in to see him, I found that the family had not exaggerated. Here was a man just wanting to die.

I asked them whether they had ever given him a drink. They said he had been a teetotaler all his life. Therefore they had hesitated to offer it to him.

I started him off on an ounce of port wine before dinner. Within a few days he was eating better than he had in months. Then I ordered—as if I were suggesting he take pills—a tablespoonful of brandy four times a day. Like a miracle drug, it transformed him within 48 hours into an acceptable member of the family—full of his old enthusiasms and talkative and cheerful.

I have seen scores of similar reactions in the elderly to judicious use of alcohol. The late Dr. E. J. Stieglitz backs up my opinion in writing: "It is of considerable assistance in the management and control of arteriosclerotic changes in elderly persons—. Alcohol is often most constructive in increasing vigor and endurance in the elderly."

Keep remembering this if you have an unhappy, unmanageable oldster in your family. Although alcohol is no cure-all, it is certainly worth a try before filling up the patient with many varieties of tranquilizers—which often disturb the patient more than they help.

What Type of Drinker Are You?

If you drink, it is wise to step off and take an honest look at yourself. In what class do you belong? If you are not a teetotaler you are one of three: 1. a social drinker who can take it or leave it. 2. An excessive drinker who drinks much more and **thinks** he can take it or leave it. 3. A chronic alcoholic.

As I have indicated earlier, I believe that there are thousands of teetotalers above the age of forty who would be better off if they drank moderately. This is especially true if they are abnormally tense and already are suffering from diseases of tension. If you are over forty-five and don't take alcohol, why not ask your doctor whether or not you have any contra-indications against it. If not, and he also agrees that alcohol is often an excellent antidote to tension and anxiety, then I hope you will not refuse to take it simply on moral grounds. I have known people who classed themselves—or their friends—as alcoholics simply because they took some wine or a few tablespoonfuls of liquor before dinner. To requote: "The distorted ideas about alcohol which are commonly held among the public in general are largely founded on emotionalism."

Definition of the Social Drinker

It is not difficult to know whether or not you are a social drinker. Can you take it or leave it? If the answer is unequivocally **yes,** then you fall into the large class of over 50 million drinkers who gain rather than suffer from drinking.

If you are a social drinker you often go days and weeks without taking a drink. Often you take one only because your wife says, "You look tired, dear. You must have had a hard day. Let me fix you a highball." Having taken it, you may say that you're going to take one every night— but being a non-compulsive drinker you forget until the next time.

Perhaps you take a martini when you go out to lunch with a friend or customer. At a cocktail party you may occasionally go overboard and take two or three drinks. You have never been drunk. You have never had blackouts. You are very careful not to get behind the wheel until you have had some coffee to sober you up. Do you measure up to these standards? Then you are a social drinker and alcohol is no problem.

Coffee Not a Sure Antidote

Incidentally, in reference to "sobering up" in preparation for driving, this will interest you. And perhaps save you from an avoidable accident.

In these days when cocktail parties are the vogue—and at which people often drink more than they can safely handle, there is supposed to be one sure, universal antidote to too much liquor. I refer to coffee.

When a man has had too much and is saying goodbye to his host, it is not unusual for him to hear: "Frank, don't you think a hot cup of coffee is a good suggestion before you get behind the wheel?"

Sometimes Frank will agree; but more often he will say, "I'm all right. Forget it."

However well-meant, the suggestion to take coffee may not be a good one. I'm sorry to disillusion so many who depend upon coffee to clear the brain and sharpen the reflexes, but a question has risen whether or not a cup of coffee can transform a person who has "had a few" into a safe driver.

At least, it doesn't seem that coffee speeds recovery in rats. In experiments with laboratory rats Professors F. W. Hughes and R. B. Forney of the Indiana University Medical Center found that coffee even prolongs poor behavior in alcoholism. They found that the caffein seemed to prolong the effects, even after all traces of alcohol had disappeared from the circulation.

A rat isn't a man, and a man isn't (necessarily) a rat: nevertheless, this is timely caution. I have known many people who, having taken one too many, believed that a cup or two of coffee was the immediate and effectual answer to the problem. I recall one who insisted on driving home and got into a serious accident. Moral: coffee isn't always the answer to safety. There is a police slogan which says, "Take one for the road" (meaning a cup of coffee) if you have had a few drinks. A better slogan would be "better take a cab from a cocktail party."

Alcohol and Driving Are Dangerous Mixture

For it is unquestionably true that the man who takes alcohol before he drives is a menace to himself and to others on the road. And often it makes no difference whether the driver is a social drinker, an excessive drinker or a chronic alcoholic. In fact, often the social drinker is the greater danger because just one drink lifts up his pride in his ability to manage the car.

How do you feel when you let Junior or sister have the car for an evening? Don't you sometimes worry yourself sick, imagining all sorts of horrible accidents when they are out later than expected? Don't you picture the roads infested with drunken drivers?

Why do you think, when starting out on a long automobile journey, or even when getting into your car to drive only a few miles to your home, that friends s~ "Drive carefully, now."

Deep down in all of us, imbedded in the subconscious mind, is the realization and the fear that "the road" is an ever-present hazard to life. Thirty-eight thousand deaths a year in highway accidents and hundreds of thousands of people maimed, should keep reminding us that the automobile (especially with an alcoholic behind the wheel) is an inevitable risk to our happiness and future. The worst offender is the man or woman with a drink under the belt.

We Are Too Complacent

For years I have been beating the drums against our complacency, especially regarding the problem alcoholic behind the wheel. It was therefore, with great satisfaction that I read the following letter to *The Journal of the American Medical Association,* written by Horace E. Campbell, M.D., Chairman of the Automotive Safety Subcommittee of the Colorado State Medical Society. See if you don't agree:

Police records are replete with instances of drivers convicted again and again of driving while intoxicated. These records reveal that drivers, after an arbitrary length of time, are allowed their licenses, until finally they kill some other driver or themselves.

It is finally coming to be realized that many of these drivers are chronic alcoholics. The chronic alcoholic, or problem drinker, is completely immune to slogans. Safety campaigns do not touch him at all. Scathing lectures by judges, even terms in jail, are just water on this duck's back. He is a compulsive drinker.

Repetitive offenders should be sentenced to psychiatric investigation. Increasingly, traffic courts must have good, closely related psychiatric clinics. Detroit's Recorder's Court was the first of these and is still the best. The numbers of feeble-minded, psychotic, alcoholic, emotionally deranged, licensed drivers revealed by this clinic is appalling.

If investigation reveals a chronic alcoholic then the sentence must not be a fine or even a term in jail, but assignment to a treatment center for alcoholics. A wise judge has said that we cannot force a man to stop drinking, but we can force him to take treatment. The chronic alcoholic is now recognized as the cause of a substantial percentage of all motor accidents. In one well-controlled study, problem drinkers were the drivers in a third of the serious crashes studied. Current judicial practices in the United States are completely unrealistic as far as the chronic alcoholic driver is concerned.

Do you know what is especially sad about all this? We can blame it on our own complacency. If an aroused public in every community in the U.S.A. got up on its feet and said, "Stop this unnecessary slaughter—and we mean it," it wouldn't be long before legislators would buckle down and place this problem at the top of their agenda. Then, at last, we'd have some peace of mind whenever anyone in our family got behind the wheel of the car.

But keep remembering what I have been saying, you social drinkers. You have your responsibility, too. One drink and you must be on your guard. And please recall that the cup of coffee may not be the sure antidote, and the guarantee of safety, that you have always considered it to be.

Are You an Excessive Drinker?

Now, I presume you are still standing off trying to look at yourself objectively to see just where you fit in. Perhaps you wonder if you are an excessive drinker rather than a social drinker. See if I can help you make the diagnosis. I would label you an excessive drinker if you followed this pattern:

Often you take a swig in the morning if you have had too many the night before. You take two or three martinis at lunch every day. Often you take a bottle of ale at the time if you are having some beef. On the way home you stop off at a bar to have a few beers or highballs. When you get home you take two or three ounces of scotch or rye before dinner. Perhaps some brandy after dinner and a beer or two while watching television. When you go to a cocktail party or any other affair where celebration is in order, you will take at least a half-dozen highballs —and are proud to say that you can hold your liquor.

When family or friends say, "Don't you think you have been having too much lately?" you are quick to reply, "I can handle it all right. Never missed a day from business yet."

Man, you're an excessive drinker. And in danger of missing more than a few days of business. You are walking a tightrope that swings precariously between excessive drinking (supposedly controlled) and chronic alcoholism. The danger is inherent in the false belief that you can cut down when you want to. Remember that any severe emotional strain may topple you over into the chasm of chronic alcoholism. Worry about family, illness or financial reverses are the potential enemies waiting to spring. They can turn you into a hopelessly compulsive drinker.

Remedy Is Evident

The remedy is evident. Change from an excessive drinker to a purely social drinker—otherwise you will find that the change from a chronic alcoholic back to an excessive drinker is not so easy.

Resolve **now** to limit your alcohol intake. Take only one martini at lunch—and no beer. Only a one-or-two-ounce highball at night. Or, a bottle of beer with your dinner, instead. At cocktail parties, never take more than three drinks. Let that be your limit. If you take immediate action to remove the excess daily intake, the chances of your becoming a chronic alcoholic are remote.

Are You a Chronic Alcoholic?

Are you still standing off, looking? Do you wonder if you are a chronic alcoholic? That is usually evident to others as well as to yourself. If you have had recurring Lost Weekends and blackouts the diagnosis is easy. If

every day. That we see the human derelicts and the suffering of the innocents; that no doctor I ever knew became "hardened" against the misery the bottle causes in shattered families and "lost lifetimes."

As an example of our deep interest in the problem of chronic alcoholism I quoted from a letter just received from a Dr. S. of New Jersey, chief of the alcoholic service in a hospital there:

> We know darn well that the alcoholic is sick, and that one of the cardinal symptoms of his sickness is the dilution of his will power in a stream of alcohol. Asking such a man to stop drinking and come to his senses as we would like to see him do, is like asking a paralytic to do the twist. . . .
>
> In my humble opinion, what we need, is a more dynamic and a more sympathetic approach to chronic alcoholism, as we so very well manifest to the leukemic, to the cancerous or to the paralytic. Though we do not know exactly what makes a person alcoholic, we do know that frustration and all kinds of pressures—emanating through economical, social, familial, emotional misadventures—have a great deal to do with it. For many a person with a low grade of tolerance towards suffering it is so easy to slumber under the wings of alcohol.
>
> Until a breakthrough comes, and it will come, I am sure (a great deal of research is underway) let us treat the alcoholic as a human being who is really sick and disabled in no less degree than one afflicted with polio or mitral stenosis. Let us have patience with these patients. We must continue to try to understand their problem and come up with sincere, practical advice and help.

Delerium Tremens No Joke

I agree with the thoughts expressed by Dr. S., and I think so do most doctors. Any physician who isn't deeply touched by what the ravages of alcohol can do to his patient and his family must be cold and steely-hearted indeed. Likewise, do I believe that the populace in general now looks upon the alcohol problem with sympathy and interest. Not too many years ago, for example, many looked upon delerium tremens (the DTs) as a joke. You remember the stories about green elephants and other bizarre creatures, common hallucinations of these to-be-pitied patients. Now, that we look upon chronic alcoholism as a disease and not just a bad habit, we realize that delerium tremens is an important enemy to overcome; it kills anywhere from 5-15 per cent of patients who suffer from it.

It usually comes on when the heavy drinker is deprived of his alcohol. It is called the "withdrawal syndrome." The patient becomes confused, has a coarse tremor and becomes excited. Sometimes he imagines he hears threatening voices. His tongue, finger, facial muscles and legs shake. Often his symptoms are worse at night. He becomes easily frightened and therefore belligerent and difficult to manage and restrain.

Before modern treatment, such a patient would be out of circulation anywhere from one to three weeks with the worst symptoms lasting about 5-7 days. With newer treatments, recovery time is greatly lessened.

The doctor's job is to try to overcome the upset in the body's metabolism and the swelling of the brain cells.

Therefore, he gives large amounts of vitamins (especially the B complex group), sugar solution by vein, drugs to bring down the brain swelling, magnesium, tranquilizers as needed, fluids containing electrolytes (important minerals) and cortisone-type medicine.

The Good and Bad of Alcohol

I keep giving you this gruesome side of the alcohol picture so you will know I haven't lost sight of its potential menace. But it gives me the springboard to keep reminding you that the person who reaches middle-age without having become an alcoholic will probably not ever face the real problems I have outlined.

It is the teenager or the college student; or the man in his late twenties or thirties trying to hold his own in the mad swim to keep his head above business or professional waters; or the youngster (married or single, male or female) beset by unbearable tensions in home life: such are the ones who need to guard themselves against the spectre of chronic alcoholism.

There are the susceptible people, and what causes their susceptibility to alcohol habituation we do not know. Is it a psychosis? A psychoneurosis? A nutritional deficiency? An inability to withstand stress? An imbalance in the glands? Whatever the cause, it usually shows up early in life; by the time you are 40, I think you are safe to take alcohol as a daily ration.

My opinion, based on experience in the front lines of medical practice, continues to be that there are many middle-aged and elderly people in this world who—bereft of alcohol for one reason or another—are actually doing themselves a disservice in being abstainers.

For thousands of years—in spite of its potential for harm—alcohol has brought mankind relaxation and pleasure. It will continue to do so until eternity, for man will never give up the "grape" or "honey" or "potato"—or whatever means he has to make an innocuous foodstuff by fermentation into the "aqua vitae."

Summary of Chapter

1. Don't agree that your children may drink at an early age.
2. Alcohol can be a boon or a poison.
3. People rarely become alcoholics after 40.
4. Alcohol is usually interdicted in those who have extremely high blood pressure, ulcer, gall bladder disease, gout, kidney or liver disease; and especially in those who are emotionally unstable.
5. Doctors know the grief alcohol can cause.
6. Alcohol helps cut the rope of tension.
7. Alcohol helps calm the aged.
8. The problem of alcoholism goes back a few million years.
9. The anti's and the pro's have been at each other for years.
10. Alcohol helps many angina patients.
11. Are you a teetotaler? A social drinker? An excessive drinker? A chronic alcoholic? A frank and honest answer is essential.
12. Coffee isn't always effective as an antidote for intoxication in preparation for driving.

13. We have been too complacent in battling the danger of intoxicated drivers.
14. Alcohol is of value for those over 40.
15. Delerium tremens is no joke.
16. Nevertheless, man will never give up his alcoholic beverages.

The FOURTH Commandment: Thou Shalt Not Take Alcohol

Forget it IF:

1. You are over 40 and are not now an alcoholic.
2. You have angina or other evidence of coronary disease.
3. You find you require more and more tranquilizers.
4. You refuse to take alcohol only on "moral" grounds.

———

NOTE:

Many over 40 who do not take alcohol might be better off if they did.

Remember it IF:

1. You are a teenager.
2. You are under 40. Take it with caution.
3. You are emotionally unstable.
4. You have very high blood pressure.
5. You have ulcer or gout.
6. You have liver or kidney disease.
7. You expect to be behind the wheel of a car.

———

NOTE:

If you take alcohol in spite of warnings by your doctor you may actually be committing slow suicide.

5

Thou shalt not
Eat Too Much?

You don't have to eliminate the foods you like from your diet in order to lose weight.

"*Dr. Steincrohn,* I have been sick for 13 years with high blood pressure, slight heart trouble, dropsy and arthritis. I have always been overweight since childhood. I am 56 years old, and as you can see, very much overweight. I have tried to take it off by dieting, but can't seem to lose any weight.

"I have asked my doctor to give me pills to help me take off weight, but he tells me he cannot because of my high blood pressure which sometimes goes up to 300. I had a slight stroke which sometimes affects my eye, and makes it blurry at times.

"He sent me to you for another opinion. I hope you agree that it's all right for me to take the pills. Otherwise I don't see how I can curb my appetite. I had a metabolism test and the doctor says my thyroid is all right.

"I want so bad to lose some weight as my arthritis is so bad. If some weight was taken off maybe I could walk better. My knee is bad and keeps on aching. I get out of the house only if somebody takes me out for a ride in the car.

"I just lost my husband and two sisters and I get very nervous and cry so much. If I could walk I could get out more often and I am not lazy and I like to do my housework but at times I cannot even do that.

"About ten years ago a doctor put me on a diet and gave me pills to help reduce. I lost a lot of weight—although I admit it came back after a few months. I'd like to try again. That's why I hope you say taking the reducing pills is all right."

Not All Patients Can Take "Reducing Pills"

This patient's imploring request points up a number of problems that may be beneficial to many others. First, the problem of obesity. She has had this condition since childhood. Now, at 56, she is again anxious to lose weight. It's the old story of locking the barn after the horses have been stolen. Although I believe that weight loss at this stage might still help her physical condition, ten or twenty years ago was the better time for treating her obesity.

Very often doctors have good reasons for not prescribing anti-fat drugs. Although amphetamine and its family members are often prescribed for patients who have high blood pressure complicating obesity, I believe this lady should be one of the exceptions. She didn't like it when I told her that the history of heart trouble, dropsy and a possible recent stroke certainly seemed to make inadvisable the use of any of these reducing drugs.

The patient's problem brings up another point—that of

doctor-patient relationship. Although I told her that her doctor was using good judgment in refusing to allow her to take appetite-depressing drugs, she persisted in asking for such medication. Being human, doctors are sometimes "broken down" by a patient's requests. Against their good judgment they may give in.

For example, a doctor will sometimes allow a patient back to work earlier than he should, because of the patient's insistence. Or, the other way around, allow him to stay home when he should be back at work. Another time the doctor may suggest x-rays and the patient will have the doctor postpone them for some reason or other. Often, harm comes to the patient because of the time lost.

So I again suggested to our obese lady that, being unhappy about her arthritis and other physical discomforts, the safest and best procedure was to follow her doctor's advice: no pills but weight reduction by diet alone. I told her that if she were my patient I would most certainly advise against the use of drugs to curb her appetite. She would have to rely on will power.

But the real lesson here is this: the time to treat obesity is early in life—long before complications have set in.

No Secret for Weight Reduction

Patients often ask: "What is the key to the secret of weight reduction? Why do some persons have to work hard at it to lose an ounce? Others seem to shed weight so easily."

I tell them that there is no secret key. Losing weight is as simple as 2 plus 2 makes 4. It's simply a matter of intake of calories and outgo of energy. Eat less than your body needs to sustain you and you will waste away. However, if you cut down the excess calories to a normal intake, then you will stay in normal weight-balance.

Patients say: "What you say is logical. We agree. But everybody knows that! What we'd like is the secret. Just one hint that will assure weight loss in those of us who have been unable to lose."

The answer is so obvious you will probably discard it as being unimportant. Yet, here it is. I give it to you as the prime necessity or essential in successful weight reduction. If you really want to lose, you must first instill deep in yourself the **will to lose.**

Sounds ridiculous doesn't it? You will say, "Of course everybody who wants to lose has the will to lose. Otherwise why should we even think of going on a diet?"

However, in my practice I have found this to be true: there is a distinction between the superficial and deep desire to melt off those pounds. Most people who decide to go on a diet make only a superficial effort to do so. Therefore, they quit at the end of a day, a week, a month, three to six months—or postpone going on a diet at all. "I'll start tomorrow" is the universal, wavering resolve.

Many people who take off twenty or thirty pounds are like chronic alcoholics. After a few months they fall off the wagon. In a matter of weeks they fatten up again.

Why Pounds Accumulate

The reason? Their *will to lose* has disintegrated. People who want to lose—yet haven't a strongly developed will to lose—give many reasons for their repeated failures in reduction. Week after week they will return without having lost an ounce. In fact, often they gain while on a reduction regime.

For example, cooks have told me they have observed their diets carefully. Therefore, they can't understand why they haven't lost. They say (and seem to believe it): "I guess my weight comes from breathing in the food odors in the kitchen."

Likewise, other patients will swear they eat very little. They can't understand why the weight gradually keeps accumulating. "I only have orange juice for breakfast and tea and toast for lunch. I just can't figure it out," they say.

Then you talk to them some more and you uncover clues that they were perhaps unaware of. For example, some eat little until the hours between 6 P.M. and midnight. A large dinner plus television refreshments and midnight snacks easily counterbalances the effects of low calorie breakfasts and lunches.

Calories Find Their Way

I think you will agree that when the will isn't there, the calories have a way of finding their entrance. Cocktail parties, dinner celebrations, weddings, bachelor parties, lodge meetings, bridge club affairs and dozens of other "outside-the-house-filling-stations"—such are the methods obesity uses in its all-out attack on us food-loving human beings. Add the anxieties and tensions which so many have, as a cause of their constant nibbling and overeating, and you have another important factor in the obesity problem.

As I am subject to these same temptations, I know how difficult it is to abstain from eating too much. I know that dieting is "no picnic." Nevertheless, I have given you the secret many of you asked for. If you nurture and develop within you a steel-hard core of the **will to lose,** you will be able to forego all dietary indiscretions. The result is you won't gain. You can forget that heredity or "glands" have anything to do with the common garden-variety of obesity.

I received a letter from a former patient who now lives in California. She said: "Isn't the urge to overeat a sickness? Isn't it true that some people are unable to resist a second helping—as others can't resist a third or fourth martini or highball?

Need for a National a.a.

"My point is this: A.A. (Alcoholics Anonymous) has been doing a wonderful job in reclaiming alcoholics. Why can't we have a similar organization designated by the small letters a.a. (adiposity anonymous)?

"If in union there is strength—it must be especially true for weak-willed people, who through no fault of their own, cannot resist food. I have heard of such clubs, but I understand that most are on a local rather than on a national scale.

"I wish that you would some time publicize the need for such a national organization. If you can be the 'spark' of a national a.a. you will have done much for the health of the country. I recall how often you mentioned the dangers of obesity when I used to visit you."

When I replied to her letter, I told her to consider me on her side. I hope we can enlist as many enthusiastic people as a national a.a. deserves. Although I agree that using the small letters a.a. distinguishes the proposed organization from Alcoholics Anonymous (A.A.), if I had my way I'd use oversized A's to indicate the relative importance of obesity and chronic alcoholism. Of the two, obesity is potentially more dangerous. For in the shadow of obesity flourish such life-shortening conditions as high blood pressure, diabetes, cancer, accidents, arteriosclerosis, coronary thrombosis, arthritis and many other killers.

Yet, I'll settle on the lower case a.a. if potential members will remember that the small letters do not imply that obesity is less important.

Many Anti-Obesity Clubs

There are many local anti-obesity clubs. A number of years ago I spoke with an enthusiastic member of the Manchester, Conn. Wates Club. You cannot join unless your application for membership is filled by a physican. Incidentally, doctors come in to talk to members about heart disease, cancer and other conditions.

Meetings are held every Tuesday. This is serious business. Your "weight for the week" is not considered "legal" unless ascertained by two official weighers and duly recorded. I understand that "thousands of pounds" have been lost by members of this organization. (Its president lost 49 pounds during her year's term of office.)

The member who loses the most gets a free trip to Bermuda. Members must pay 25 cents for each pound gained. But what's even worse, non-losing members are herded off by themselves (during meetings) to the "Pig-

Pen." Here they sit quietly—unable to talk to one another without risking expulsion.

At that time the Manchester Wates Club had about 130 members and the meetings were well attended. I asked my informant how many lose weight. About three quarters of the members do.

"Do you think," I asked her, "that your 'Pig-Pen' will ever be empty during meetings?"

She answered: "Human nature being what it is, **That'll Be The Day.**

TOPS (Take Off Pounds Sensibly) is an organization with chapters in several states. These and many other clubs are doing good work in eliminating excess poundage and promoting better health in the United States. Nevertheless, I believe there's a real need—and I was never more serious—for a national a.a. In one way or another we must instill the **will to lose.**

Have you tried reducing and failed? Perhaps what you need is the helping hand of a neighbor who has at last succeeded. Many patients have told me "I'm sure if I belonged to such a club I would be determined to stick on a diet for my health's sake and also to improve my appearance."

I have known many "hopelessly fat" patients who at last overcame their obesity when they joined a club to fight the common enemy. For years they had been fighting alone; but the result was always failure.

Any method that is sane and harmless and will produce good results in weight loss is not to be laughed down. I know a number of colleagues who say to an obese patient: "If you haven't the stamina and will power to reduce, then you don't deserve to lose. You can join a reducing club—but I think it is silly and worthless."

An Individual Problem

I will qualify that. I believe that it is prima~ily an individual problem; that obesity is serious enough to deserve a personal, frontal attack. However, if someone has tried for months to reduce—and from psychological or other reasons fails—then he or she deserves the comfort and instillation of confidence that others likewise afflicted can supply.

I know many patients who owe their "obesity cure" to an anti-adiposity club rather than to me. Alcoholics Anonymous was at first disparaged and ridiculed by some. But its merits in the cure of chronic alcoholism are accepted now by laymen and physicians alike. I believe that its younger brother a.a. (anti-adiposity) can serve as well in the field of obesity. But, having started your club remember that your own success in reducing will depend primarily upon your own **will to lose.**

Learning all the principles of your new club is the easiest part of it.

What you will have to learn is how to pass your refrigerator door without grabbing its handle every time you have the urge "for just a little snack." Whether you join a club or not—dieting is an intensely personal crusade against fat.

From what I have been saying it is evident that I recognize obesity as an enemy. I consider it as the beginning of disease itself in many conditions. There is no question that you can't be fat and fit at the same time. It is true that obesity is life-shortening. Nevertheless, I do not always go along with the commandment: **Thou Shalt Not Gain Weight.**

Don't Change Signals After 70

For example, consider Mrs. K., aged 75 who is concerned about herself because she is getting fat. She is 5'4" and weighs about 200 pounds.

> "I went to a doctor for weight control," she said. "He gave me some expensive green pills. They didn't help. I called him and he gave me a shot and that took a few pounds off but he said he could do no more. He didn't know what else to give me.
>
> "I eat very little but it all goes to fat. I have gained ten pounds since I stopped my treatment. I called my doctor about it and he said it was all up to me and that no doctor could lose for a patient; that it was the patient's own job to do.
>
> "And he warned me to take off the excess fat or it would go to my heart. Can you tell me what to do, Dr. Steincrohn? I am living on a social security pension and have no money for doctor bills. Please help."

The longer one has been in practice the more certain one becomes that there is no blanket rule for treating patients. We soon learn—at least we should—that each patient is a peculiarly individual problem. Although diagnostic procedures may be similar in patients, treatment differs and depends upon the patient's personality, physical and emotional make-up—and upon his age.

For example, consider again Mrs. K. Here is an apparently healthy 75-year-old lady whose only problem is obesity. What to do? We know that excess fat is bad for people. I suppose we should go about treating her intensively to take off some of those extra pounds. But wait. Is that really the wise thing to do for Mrs. K.?

Doctors differ. Perhaps most would say: "Obesity is obesity. Excess weight should come off wherever we find it."

I have felt otherwise. I have always been wary of "rigid weight enforcement" in anyone who has proved he could live until 70—fat or thin.

Don't Tamper with Nature

I have hesitated to tamper with a kindly Nature that has given a person his biblical heritage of years. I would never put anyone 70-plus on a reducing diet whether he or she was 10 or a 100 pounds overweight. My reason? Experience has taught me that conservatism is best. I would hate to upset the applecart.

In my memory stand out many apparently well, older, obese patients who went downhill rapidly and died after being put on rigid reducing regimes. It seems to me like "throwing a wrench into the machinery." Why tamper with a healthy, smooth-running 70-year-old machine that has proved itself by its good performance?

I recall the mother of a boyhood friend whose weight and measurements were almost identical with those of Mrs. K. At the time I saw her she was 81 years old and complaining of "rheumatism." She had nine wonderfully devoted children and each one thought she should be put on a reducing diet. But at last I convinced the lot of them that she was one of the few who became old in spite of her excess weight. Why not leave well enough alone, I said. They reluctantly agreed.

A few aspirin tablets controlled her rheumatic pains due to osteoarthritis. She lived comfortably—excess weight and all—until the age of 90.

If you are young, the way to get old is to be within normal weight limits. By all means: reduce.

If you are over 70 and fat, you are an exception; because the fat usually die young. But don't let anybody talk you into reducing at this stage of the game. Change of signals may lose it for you. I believe that we doctors would make a serious mistake in treating **all** patients by rule. If that were possible, we would not have to go through so many years of training to diagnose and treat our patients. All that would be necessary would be to take out a little "rule book" from a back pocket, thumb it through to page so-and-so and have the answer to our problem.

Individual Treatment Essential

It doesn't work that way. Each obese patient—old or young—deserves specific, individual fitting of treatment to his needs and measurements. Obesity remains a stubborn challenge because of the personal element. Discovering the underlying cause is important. Is it due to psychological causes like inner tension and anxiety? Then two main courses are open: an investigation by family physician or psychiatrist and appropriate treatment. In many patients I have seen weight-loss for the first time after they were allowed to "ventilate" (get things off their chest) and after they took tranquilizers to "detensify." Not until then was it possible to put the **will to lose** into effect.

Is the weight increase due to the habit of taking second and third portions? The remedy is evident.

Is it due to lack of exercise? Here, too, the remedy is evident. But remember that exercise is also a personal thing. Some can sit all day, eat well and still be normal-weighted. Others pile on the pounds unless they get out of that chair once in a while.

Is it snacks? As I said to one woman who had gained tremendously because she not only ate three large meals, but kept nibbling at snacks most of the day: "Why not try just living on snacks and giving up your regular meals?" Not realizing I was joking, that is just what she did for a month. For the first time in years she returned to the office with a deficit of about 16 pounds. Finally, she was able to put the horse before the cart: she ate her regular meals and gave up the snacks. In her case, tranquilizers and an explanation of the reasons for her tensions were the dominant factors in her improvement.

I have known hundreds of patients who could not begin to lose until they took amphetamine drugs for a few weeks to decrease their appetite. Others did well on tranquilizers alone. Still others required a combination of amphetamines and tranquilizers. However, it is important—when using such combinations—not to give too large doses of tranquilizers. In many patients such treatment decreases the effectiveness of the appetite-decreasing amphetamines.

I have written often on the need to diet, the dangers of obesity, and how the job can be done. Having treated thousands of overweight persons, I am certainly aware that, for some, dieting is an almost unsurmountable obstacle.

Some Don't Have the Will Power

They just don't have the stamina—or will power—to fight off the calories. That is why there are so many failures in the struggle against the extra pounds. Here, for example, is a letter from Mrs. D., in Indiana, which shows how some people have to struggle with their excess weight.

> "*Dear Dr. Steincrohn:* Perhaps we fat slobs do not deserve any sympathy; however, I think many neglect to mention the psychological (real or unreal) need some overweight people have for their excessive eating habits.
>
> "After listening to my mother's fairy tales of how the weight 'would some day go away' I was lucky enough to realize the true facts when I was a teen-ager. No, the weight doesn't just go away. I know I eat a lot and enjoy eating.
>
> "Perhaps the saddest thing about dieting is this. It becomes eternal!
>
> "I lost weight in college—all the way down to 155. (I'm at 195 now.) After that daily sacrifice I found some pleasure in the slim shadow of my former self. But the joy was short-lived. To maintain that 155 pounds meant never to eat again—well, at least, not the way I enjoy it. Healthful torture, is, unfortunately, a slow torture when the poor victim sees little of the delight but plenty of the torment. Give us slobs our psychological due. Signed, FATSO."

In reply I told this unhappy woman to stop calling herself **Slob and Fatso** and stop feeling so sorry for herself —and to get down to the business of dieting, even if it hurts. Nevertheless, I couldn't get away from the feeling that there is something about the problem of obesity which we doctors don't even suspect. Something deep and evasive.

I have often said that obesity is the beginning of serious disease. Perhaps I should say that obesity is disease itself. It strikes some and spares others. Why? We don't think it is glandular? We don't think it is hereditary? We believe only that it is due to an excessive intake of calories. And this belief is the reason for the myriads of diets that spring up everywhere to control weight gain.

Obesity Still a Mystery

But the prime question is why some gain and others don't! One reason advanced is that there is a disturbance of an appetite center in that part of the brain called the hypothalamus. But what causes the disturbance? And exactly what kind of disturbance is it? Why does it cause people of great will and determination in other departments of their lives to become actual weaklings in their abnormal craving for food?

One sees an attractive food ad on TV and is sent running for the refrigerator to "stoke up"; while another looks at it complacently and does not feel the urge to eat.

One looks at a TV ad of beer and also runs for the refrigerator to open a can; another looks on unaffected.

One sees the TV spiel and listens to the announcer who lights up his favorite brand of cigarette. Unconsciously he feels in his pocket for his pack and lights up; while another looks on unaffected.

What is there in us human beings that makes one fat, another an alcoholic, and the third a chain-smoker? As is commonly said: "Each to his own poison." But why?

Although doctors talk much about the dangers of obesity, I do not think that we have dug deeply enough to find the answer to its cause. I doubt that as much money is being spent on research in this field as is spent in less-important, more highly publicized illnesses. Some day we must come up with an unevasive answer to the simple question put by so many who are overweight: "Why is it that my friend Joe can eat all he wants and not put on an extra once, while I have to struggle on a starving diet to take off a pound or two?"

Frying Pan or Fire?

Or, be able to understand such common problems like the following:

> "*Dr. Steincrohn,* my husband is 52 years old, about six feet tall and up until recently weighed around 155 pounds. About two years ago he gave up smoking because of a morning cough. His coughing stopped but he put on about 30 pounds. Some of this extra weight has gone to his waistline, neck, shoulders and the usual places for his age. However, I'd say that about two-thirds of it has settled in a large, bloated 'pot.' Otherwise his health is good. My question is this: shall he take up cigarette smoking again to lose?"

In effect here is what I told her: you mean it's a case of the frying pan or the fire. Too much smoking isn't good; neither is too much eating, and the subsequent weight-gain. It is not uncommon for some people to put on a few pounds after they have given up cigarettes. I guess it's because their taste-buds are in better shape and their enjoyment of food produces a better appetite. However, some people use this as an excuse—somehow believing that if they give up one bad habit they deserve some kind of repayment by indulging too much in something else.

I told her: As I see it, your husband must choose between a cigarette cough and something much more serious. If he continues to gain, he invites the complications which so many obese people are heir to: gall bladder trouble, high blood pressure, coronary disease, diabetes and lesser discomforts. Tell him that he deserves a pat on the back for overcoming the cigarette habit; but he will be doubly smart if he uses the same will power to curb his appetite. Of the two, I think that obesity is the greater danger. But that doesn't mean he needs to take up smoking again.

As I look back upon that oversimplification of the problem, I realize that it's easy to sit atop a comfortable chair and look down and give oracular advice, knowing full well that something important is missing in our knowledge about obesity. But I am not conscience-stricken, any more than I am in our helplessness in not yet finding the real cause of cancer or arteriosclerosis. We have to work with the weapons we have at hand and do the best we can until the bright light of truth shines upon these problems.

Temporarily, our greatest weapon against obesity is **diet.** For many this word has all the bad connotations of all four-letter words concentrated into the worst one of all: **diet.** Taking away food from the obese person is like taking away liquor or dope from other addicts. Yet, if weight-loss there is to be, only dieting will accomplish it.

Not in Favor of Crash Diets

I don't believe in crash diets. People who go in for these new-formula diets are usually more interested in the rate of weight loss than in their health. A safe guess is that the underlying motivation for taking off those pounds is improvement of looks.

Most often they do not realize that "self-treatment of obesity" can be overdone to the special detriment of heart, kidney, diabetes and high blood pressure patients.

Ideally, weight loss should be a slow, steady thing. Rapid loss followed by rapid gain—when repeated often over a period of years—can actually be very harmful. I think it's better to stay fat than go "up and down-up and down" like an elevator that has gone beserk. This whipping of the body's metabolism certainly doesn't do the major organs of the body any good. Slow unhurried reduction, by eating the usual foods, in lesser amounts, is the ideal way.

If you are many pounds overweight, call in your doctor to help you. With many patients, I worked as hard trying to slow the rate of their weight loss. I asked them, "What's your hurry? It has taken you years to put it on; take your time losing. Besides, it will stay off longer."

You have guessed it—I am opposed to short cuts in dieting. Originally, only one or two companies had the lucrative 900-calorie diet field to themselves. Now, there are more than 100 companies selling the "magic" diet in liquid or powder form. When so many competitors rock the boat, it invariably sinks.

Although these formulas are supposed to have all the necessary minerals, vitamins, proteins, fats and carbohydrates—something is necesarily missing. If nature didn't intend us to bite and chew many varieties of food stuffs, I doubt that she would have provided us with teeth!

Why the Hurry?

To repeat, go slow. There's no hurry. In fact, if you have complications like diabetes or atherosclerosis, it's definitely essential to go slow in weight loss.

If you are only a few pounds over, you can do it all by yourself. You don't need a doctor; you do not need a fast-acting 900-calorie regime. Remember you can't stay on it all your life. And when you go off it, and back to your regular diet again, it is inevitable you will gain.

Some time ago I watched a pharmacist wait for a stout woman to make up her mind between buying a reducing formula containing banana or chocolate flavor. After 15 minutes' hesitancy she decided upon the chocolate.

Recently I asked the same druggist how the 900-calorie diets were doing. He said: "Still selling, but they've slowed up quite a bit. People are tired of diet fads. But I'm not worrying. They'll be back in droves when the next diet fad sweeps the country."

I agree. I predict that within a few months or years a new crash diet will sweep the country like a contagion. People will forget all about the present "reducing-champ." They will go ga-ga about the new formula—and spend millions in hard-earned money to pay for it. What a loss! And not necessarily a permanent weight-loss!

Council Statement

You will be interested in some points made by the Council on Foods and Nutrition, of the American Medical Association. They appear in a Council Statement which I received:

—Individuals who are excessively overweight and who may have additional ailments such as heart disease, kidney disease, or diabetes should not undertake weight reduction without medical guidance.

—A therapeutic formula diet is a preparation which in no way resembles the obese individual's ordinary diet. Consequently, the obese subject is unable to appreciate the difference in food composition between the formula and his ordinary diet. Furthermore, monotony of the formula diet may result in its abandonment after a short period.

The formula per se is certainly not a panacea for obesity.

Weight reduction should be achieved without the use of crash diets or bizarre preparations. Only the dietary program which results in permanent weight loss and lifetime control of weight will be a satisfactory one.

Philip L. White, Sc.D., Secretary, Council of Foods and Nutrition, American Medical Association, added: "Extensive weight reduction should be carried out only with a physician's guidance, and with diets which are tailored to the individual's needs. Weight reduction must be considered a long-term procedure and education of the individual to the faults of his past eating habits is essential. Only the dietary program which results in permanent weight loss and lifetime control of weight will be a satisfactory one."

And yet, the wonder diets continue to sprout and flourish on the American way of life every few years. They come from nowhere and go nowhere, leaving in their wake emptier pockets, empty gratification and no permanent loss of weight in most cases. Temporarily they stimulate the imaginations of women who see their future sylphlike figures; and of men who think they will look like Don Juans. The diets cause much excitement and fluttering and are then gone forever—until another one comes along. They are come and gone like a comet. Anyone can concoct a diet which is likely to sweep the country. From personal experience I know that when you deal with diets, you become immersed in the emotions of people— not with their minds. The most intelligent may become the most obtuse.

The Blue Grape Diet

A number of years ago—while a silly diet craze was enveloping the United States—I attempted to neutralize the excitement by creating a diet of my own. I called it **The Blue Grape Diet**—the diet to end all diets! I under-lined the fact that it was a ridiculous contrivance whose only purpose was to put some sense into people's heads.

I won't give you the complete diet here, because—as I shall show later—doing so would only defeat its very purpose. But in the main it consisted of 7 blue grapes at each meal accompanied by water, vitamins, egg yolk, skimmed milk, toasted crackers, raisins, almonds, cottage cheese, coffee, and steak. Eight raisins, 3 almonds and 7 blue grapes—that was the basic requirement! Does the inclusion of steak interest you? I recommended this silly portion: one inch, by three-quarters inch, by one-half inch. (Quite a mouthful!)

I also added the following ridiculous suggestions: For those who so desire, you may have two stalks of celery to be taken 15 minutes before retiring. You must weigh yourself at 2:30 A.M. twice weekly (wearing only your left bedroom slipper at the time)! I also added that if you awake in the early morning hours feeling famished it is permissible to peel three (white) grapes and wash them down with one-half glass of vichy water.

This, then, was my diet to end all diets. I promised that if you would endure this diet faithfully you would lose weight steadily. In fact, if you never returned to a sensible diet, you would soon waste away to the bone—if some other infection didn't get you down in the interim.

I emphasized that I had tried to conceive my diet in such a manner that it would be as preposterous, lopsided and nonsensical as possible. That in principle it did not differ from such former champions as the 11-day diet, the 28-day diet, the "Hollywood diet," the banana diet, the apple-pear-peach diet, and many others.

And I ended it all by asking: "How silly can we get?"

It seems that to make any formula the talk of the country all you need to do is just add a few figs here, one radish there; or one green banana and three or four string beans.

After My Book Was Published

After my book was published came the reader reactions. From all over the United States came such questions, written in all seriousness:

"Do you have to peel the blue grapes, too?"

"I don't have house slippers. Is it necessary to weigh yourself with one on? Suppose I allow ¼ pound?"

"Suppose you eat the white of the egg with the egg yolk?"

"That portion of steak is mighty small! Was that a mistake in the printing?"

In thinking it over carefully, I have resolved never again to fashion a ridiculous diet in the attempt to end all silly diets. As you can see, there is always the possibility that my **Blue Grape Diet,** or even something sillier, has the potential of becoming the next wonder diet in store for the United States. I shudder to think of my responsibilities in this matter. Therefore I shall never again attempt to fight fire with fire.

The "Secret" in Dieting

It is human to look for short cuts. Unfortunately, the secret in dieting is there is no "secret." Full belief in this concept is the surest antidote against the recurring diet formulae which promise to make dieting a "pleasure."

In practice I have made it a point not to write out any diets or hand out any printed forms to help dieters. The only exceptions have been in such conditions as diabetes, high blood pressure, heart disease—and in other specific indications. Even in these patients, the common sense approach is usually the most successful one.

Common Sense Approach

Here is, in essence, the common sense approach to the problem:

1. The basis is "cutting down on" and "not eliminating" the usual foods.
2. Your doctor will tell you what are the basic requirements in proteins, fats, carbohydrates, fluids and vitamins.
3. If tension and emotional problems are a factor in in-

creased weight, proper evaluation and use of tranquilizers are helpful in dieting.
4. Your doctor will decide if you need amphetamines,
   which are appetite-depressing drugs. My feeling is that
   most people can get along without them.
5. Here is what I mean by "cut-down" instead of "cut-
   out." First, no second-helpings. If you have been ac-
   customed to six slices of bread daily, cut down to three;
   four pats of butter, down to two; two malted milks,
   down to one; a large portion of pie à la mode down to
   a half-portion. And so down the line.

If you are overweight, try this simple, unadorned
method first. I guarantee it will produce results. If there
is any "secret" to dieting, this is it: Cut *down* instead of cut
out! In my experience the best results have followed this
method. It is merely a slight change in already formed
eating habits. There is no need to learn a new regime—
which most dieters tire of, anyway. Continuing the same
foods which you have had in the past does not cause remorse and irritability as most diets do. You will still be
having most of the foods which are restricted in other
diets. Your friends will not be able to understand how you
have lost weight, yet continue to eat butter, ice cream,
desserts, gravies, bread, pies and other fattening foods.
The answer is simple. Less of the same foods, less calories.
And less calories, less weight.

Thou shalt not eat too much? Remember this commandment if you have to; forget it if you can. In either case,
the remedy is simpler than you think.

Summary: Chapter 5.

1. Don't put off weight-reduction until chronic illness takes hold. The time to treat obesity is early.
2. Amphetamines (appetite-depressants) cannot be safely used by all patients.
3. Patients sometimes influence their doctor to go against his better judgment.
4. There is no secret key to weight reduction.
5. For successful dieting you must develop the **will to lose.**
6. Like A.A. (Alcoholics Anonymous) perhaps a national a.a. (adiposity anonymous) is one answer to the obesity problem.
7. You can't be fat and fit. Obesity is the beginning of disease—perhaps a disease in itself.
8. People over 70 need not change their dietary habits even if they are overweight. Don't tamper with Nature.
9. Each obese patient deserves individual, specific treatment.
10. Each to his own poison. One becomes obese, another an alcoholic, and another a chain-smoker. Or, possibly, one becomes a "three-in-one."
11. Crash diets are ineffectual in the long run.
12. Dieting should be slow and steady.
13. Reread the ingredients of my **Blue Grape Diet.** How silly can one get?
14. Review the common sense approach to dieting.

The FIFTH Commandment: Thou Shalt Not Eat Too Much

Forget it IF:

1. You are over 70 and apparently in good health.

———

NOTE:

Don't tamper with Nature. Elderly people who are put on strict diets often begin to deteriorate.

Remember it IF:

1. You are young. Prevention of disease is more important than cure—and often easier.
2. You have diabetes.
3. You have arteriosclerosis.
4. You have high blood pressure.
5. You have arthritis.
6. You have coronary artery disease.
7. You have a history of vascular disease in your family (coronary thrombosis, angina pectoris, high blood pressure, stroke, or kidney disease).

———

NOTE:

Often the simplest and surest way to shackle the killers is by preventing or overcoming obesity.

6

Thou shalt not
Have Anxiety?

You can learn to worry less and enjoy life more.

You hear so much about nervousness and read so much about it, I suppose you wonder at times if the subject isn't being overdone.

"Wherever I go," said an acquaintance the other day, "all I hear is that so-and-so is having a nervous breakdown, that so-and-so is just plain nervous. For pity's sake, doctor, aren't there any 'normal' people left in the world? Take me, for example. Nothing seems to bother me at this time and I don't know what nerves are. But I'm wondering if I'm next. Nobody seems to escape."

Two Large Groups

I told him there are two large groups of nervous people. In the first are those who seem to be otherwise healthy. You examine them carefully and find no evidence of organic disease. Their heart, kidneys, blood pressure, liver, blood and other organs are doing an adequate job. Yet, they are nervous.

In the second group, which is often overlooked, are the people who have definite physical abnormalities. A man comes down with a coronary attack. He may show his nervousness and anxiety during the first week or two by having uncontrollable crying spells. Afterwards, he seems to be all right. Or, another is told he has tuberculosis. Another that he has sugar in his urine.

We doctors sometimes forget that these people begin to worry about themselves. They may not tell us—they are outwardly calm—but inwardly they seethe with anxiety. Such people have an "overlay" of emotional upset. Their nervousness becomes a part of their organ illness.

Therefore, both the doctor and his patient have their jobs cut out for them. If you ever become sick, don't hesitate to tell your doctor how anxious you may have become. If you don't tell him, you may befuddle and confuse him.

For example, if you have coronary disease, your pains may not actually be angina pains. Yet, you are so scared that you won't walk much, because you have heard that exertion brings on the pains. The next time you go to your doctor you may tell him that you have been having difficulty in walking. As a result, he may become suspicious of angina, whereas your trouble may be anxiety and nothing else.

Tell Your Doctor, Family, and Friends

In this day and age nerves are nothing to be ashamed of. Whether they are nerves due to worry about actual illness or "just plain nerves," don't hesitate to tell your doctor how you feel. Your foolish fears may not be so foolish! Get them off your chest.

Beyond doubt, the 20th century is the "nervous century." Is that unusual when you consider we all live in the shadow of the "bomb"? Each of us deserves the support of the other. Family, friends—and especially the doctor—should be sympathetic when the nervous person tries to unwind.

Each of us has a cracking point. It's just that some can tolerate more than others; in some cases the load hasn't become unbearably heavy. Therefore, let's not look with disdain or condescension on our nervous friends. You or I may be the next candidate for that widespread affliction called *nervousness*.

Age of Anxiety

We are living in an age of anxiety. Each individual must solve his problems (with help) in his own personal way.

Many of you will recognize this excellent description of the age we live in (*Time* magazine, Mar. 31, 1962). It is significant.

Anxiety shouts in the headlines, laughs nervously at cocktail parties, nags from the advertisements, speaks suavely in the board room, whines from the stage, clatters from the Wall Street ticker, jokes with fake youthfulness on the golf course and whispers in privacy each day before the shaving mirror and the dressing table.

Not merely the black statistics of murder, suicide, alcoholism and divorce betray anxiety (or that special form of anxiety which is guilt) but almost any innocent, everyday act: the limp or overhearty handshake, the second pack of cigarettes or the third martini, the forgotten appointment, the stammer in mid-sentence, the wasted hour before the TV set, the spanked child, the new car unpaid for.

The bomb in the background and anxiety in the foreground!

Many patients ask, "Just what is the difference between fear and anxiety? Aren't they two different words describing the same thing?"

Fear or Anxiety?

Loosely used, I suppose there's not much difference. But there is a difference. If you're suffering from fear you're scared about something about to happen right now. Suppose you are out in the jungle and a tiger is crouched to spring at you. I'm sure you will agree that you are not just being anxious—you are plain scared at what's liable to happen within the next few seconds. You either stand up and fight, or you run away. That's a fear reaction.

But anxiety, although similar, is an entirely different sensation. You own a tiger that you have raised since a cub. You hold a tiger by the tail in that you are always anxious that some day he may revert to his inborn jungle propensities and take a few bites out of you. This is being anxious about something that may happen in the future.

Why these precise definitions of the two terms: fear and anxiety? Because there are so many thousands of people who suffer from chronic anxiety. They live in fear of what may happen in the future.

If their heart skips they think: "Some day these skips will weaken my heart and I'll suddenly drop dead." Another with a headache day after day is certain that "some day the doctor will find a brain tumor." Or, "I'm sure this heartburn is really the beginning of stomach cancer, even though the doctor says there's nothing to worry about."

Now, it is natural for the pneumonia patient or the man with an attack of coronary thrombosis to be fearful—because he is in danger "right now." However, if the man with a coronary or any other acute medical or surgical condition keeps thinking for months and years that he hasn't really recovered, and that he's liable to be getting another attack any day, that's chronic anxiety.

If you are always worried about yourself, if you keep worrying about what is liable to happen to you in the future, admit to yourself that you are an unnaturally anxious person.

The remedy isn't easy. But rather than go through your days anxious and frightened, better find yourself a patient, sympathetic doctor whom you can lean on—especially on those days or weeks that life seems unbearable.

Anxiety Often Begins After 35

If it is true that for some life begins at 40, it is also true that hypochondria often begins, or becomes intensified, at 35. It's about that time of life that I see men with increasing paunch, sagging muscles, short wind, who for the first time say that they are afraid of heart or lung trouble. One wonders if he has coronary disease; another is suspicious of lung cancer.

Yesterday Mr. S., a man of 37, said to me, "I suddenly feel old. I wonder what's happening to me. I've noticed lately that I feel stiff all over in my joints for about a half hour after getting out of bed. Then it wears off and I feel as well as ever. What's the trouble?" In his case it was difficult to convince him that he was suffering the "normal" slow-up found in the transition from youth to middle age.

Last week a 35-year-old said he couldn't understand why he became so winded after taking two flights of stairs. "Is it my heart?" he asked. He felt relieved when all the tests showed a normal circulatory system. I told him that after he removes the excess baggage of about 30 pounds he carries around day and night he will not be so winded.

I am not trying to make old men out of people in their 30's. But let's be honest with ourselves. When we reach the middle years the heart, joints, muscles, lungs, arteries, all have quite a bit of mileage pile up. Only a super-optimist would expect a second-hand car to perform like a new one.

Are You a Grade Z Hypochondriac?

The main thing is to try not to go along in anxiety without trying to do something about it. Try not to be the Grade Z hypochondriac. He is the one who is afraid of the ground he walks on, of the food he eats, of the air he breathes, and even of the germs on any door knob that he touches. He is the one who keeps taking his own pulse, keeps sticking a thermometer in his mouth every few hours, and closely inspects his tongue in the mirror.

That's not being a happy hypochondriac. I know it isn't easy to develop a philosophy overnight that will wipe out your fears as surely as an eraser does a job on a blackboard. There is much "neurosis fodder" in the world today.

For example, in a review of R. V. C. Bodley's *In Search of Serenity,* A. Powell Davis writes: "The chief barriers to serenity, especially in America, Mr. Bodley sees as worry over self-importance and social standing, worry over financial problems and work, worry brought about by physical indulgence, worry attendant upon love and marriage, worry about politics and world affairs, and finally, worry about death."

Therefore, I keep telling people in their mid-thirties (or whatever age) who are just beginning to be aware of the normal slow-up, that they must accept rather than fight the natural physiological processes. That doesn't mean they have to curl up and die. There's much of living in the later years. The secret is to keep healthy and fit and to develop the ability to face your anxieties and fears rather than try to hide from them.

Have you ever wondered why, on some days, you felt vaguely anxious? As if something unpleasant was going to happen? You could find no cause for it. You or your family had no health or financial problems. You dug around for the reason but could not come up with it.

Effect of Weather on Anxiety

In many cases I have found that especially sensitive people are greatly affected by the weather and have never realized it. Many disbelieve that weather can cause them anxiety.

For example, I recall Mrs. D. who said, "Is it really true that weather actually affects our emotions? I'm a pretty even-tempered person myself. I feel as 'chirpy' on rainy days or humid days as I do on the best day of the year. Yet, I have some friends who tell me that rain depresses them. One gets so bad she almost cries. I tell them it's their imagination."

Nothing of the sort! Poor weather acts on some as blue mood music. It's difficult to reason with emotions. I recommend that you read a book on the subject by Dr. William F. Petersen called *The Patient and the Weather*. I think that will convince you.

But we've known about the connection for a long time. For example, let me quote from O. E. Dexter who wrote in 1899: "A writer in one of the British magazines some years ago aptly said, 'There are many persons who are simply victims of the weather. Atmospheric influences play upon them as the wind plays upon the strings of an aeolian harp, with the difference that the latter never utters discord in reply.

" 'A leaden sky weighs upon them with a crushing weight, and suggests all manner of unpleasant anticipation. Then the gloomy side of life comes out.

" 'The bitter sayings of people are remembered. The old groundwork of forgotten quarrels is remembered; uneasy questions arise with regard to the future. One gets tired of life. A sort of indefinite dread is the general mental influence.' "

Will you now have more forbearance with your family and friends who seem so sensitive to weather changes? At such times a pat on the back is more welcome to them than indifference, impatience and misunderstanding.

To quote Dexter again: "It is safe to say that high conditions of temperature and humidity, cloudy and rainy days, and for many people, high winds, are generally productive of more or less negative emotional states, while moderate and cool temperatures, low humidities, mild winds and clear, dry days are usually positive in their effects."

Impossible to Stop Worrying

Over the years hundreds of patients have said to me, "Just how does a fellow stop worrying? I'm a worry-wart. Everything bothers me. I go around borrowing trouble."

Invariably, my answer has been, "I've never yet met a normal human being who could stop worrying entirely. For that reason I never tell patients to stop. That's why I don't go along with the Commandment: *Thou Shalt Not Have Anxiety*. I ask patients to worry less—not to stop.

A few months ago I talked with a frantic woman in her middle forties. Here were some of her complaints: "Lately I'm worried about my breathing. I can't seem to fill my lungs with enough air. In addition, when I go to sleep at night I thrash around for hours not daring to close my eyes. That's because I'm worried I won't wake up in the morning. I continually worry about my husband's business, although he says he has never had it so good. When the kids come home a few minutes late I picture them in terrible accidents. I've got myself into an awful mess. I never used to be this way. I'm a changed woman."

In her case she was closer to the true diagnosis than she realized. She was passing through her menopause. A small percentage of women react like she did. As in most cases, a few estrogen pills and tranquilizers straightened her out.

Often it is not so simple to find the cause of worry and outline its treatment. I believe that anxiety, the medical term for worry, usually comes out of a combination of many factors, of which one's environment and one's personal reaction to it play a part.

Environment as a Cause

For example, consider environment. You have had your expectations set on a promotion in the office. Comes the day of decision and the job goes to a younger man who has been in the organization only a few years. Something distasteful has occurred in your environment.

Now comes the personal reaction. How will you take this setback? Upon the answer depends your future happiness. I have seen, as probably have you, many persons faced with this unpleasant predicament. Some have soured on life. Others have become anxious and difficult to live with. Many have actually become ill. Such is the soil in which hypertension, ulcers, chronic alcoholism and many other conditions grow and thrive.

It is one thing to know the cause of discomfort and another to know what to do for it. In the example mentioned, the most important factor is to face up to the problem and not to run away from it.

Two courses are open to prevent undue worry. If you are so constituted that continuing to work in that office would surely "eat you up" with worry, then it's best to be decisive and get another job.

If, however, you have become a mature person who knows how to accept reverses, you will stay on the job. You will dig in, work harder, hold no animosities and trust that next time you will get the promotion you think you deserve.

In other words, an antidote to chronic anxiety is a mature acceptance of unpleasant environmental factors. It is what is meant when one says to a disturbed friend, "Why don't you grow up? Everything will turn out all right."

However, there are many unfortunate persons who live scared—whose anxiety does not always depend upon the unpleasant things in their environment. With few exceptions, every normal human being is scared. You are, so am I, so's your neighbor, even though he may not admit it. Whether we will be able to overcome anxiety entirely is doubtful. In fact, a little fear is necessary for survival. Otherwise, we'd sit complacently at the cry of fire! We'd fearlessly stroll up to a lion and pat him on the head.

Where does it all begin? Many have a pat answer: "It's the conscious or unconscious fear of the bomb." Maybe. It has been said that fear of death may be at the core of all of man's anxieties. You can't listen to experts foretell the sudden destruction of 100 million Americans without becoming concerned. However, there's more to it than that. People were scared hundreds of years before explosives. If it was the case that they lived in peace amongst themselves, then they had other threats to their survival such as bad weather, wild animals, and other dangers in their environment.

A Theory About Anxiety

What might be another cause of our anxiety? Perhaps we got this way being born. Perhaps it is the stamp of the birth-process. The passage from the comfort and contentment in the uterus to the outside world is quite a strain, you know. Upon the mother, yes, but especially upon the infant.

Philosopher Immanuel Kant called a baby's first cry, "a cry of wrath at the catastrophe of birth."

Did you ever notice the facial expression of the newly born child? Did you ever see one with a smile? I doubt it. Long before the doctor smacks his nether end, the infant shows his distaste for having to emerge into a new, uncomfortable environment. His features are screwed up into a combination of expressions: resentment, fear, exhaustion, anger.

Any living organism resents giving up its creature comforts. Any living thing becomes frightened in a new, strange environment. And any young baby is hurt and exhausted from the mauling it receives as nature intermittently squeezes it, by powerful uterine contractions, into the turmoil of the outside world. It flinches at the sudden impact of cold hands, piercing sounds, strange odors. Once scared, forever scared.

The brain never forgets. On the clean blackboard of the infant's mind the difficult course of labor etches forever the hurts of the birth process. The fear remains in our subconscious forever. No eraser, no flips of the calendar, can completely eradicate it.

Someday I hope to make a study of the birth-history of people who live in unnatural anxiety and fear. How long was their mother's labor? Was it a difficult one? I won't be surprised to learn that people born by Caesarean section are less apt to be at the mercy of fear than those subjected to extra hours of birth trauma.

But enough of theorizing. Whatever the cause of anxiety, it is in each one of us in varying degrees. Heredity plays a part. So does environment—and growing up and growing older. Add school worries, job worries, health worries, survival worries—all make their insidious contributions to total chronic anxiety.

We Are All Hypochondriacs

In a general sense, then, let's agree that you and I are hypochondriacs. We can be hypochondriacal about other things than health. About a job. About love. About security. About having to die sometime. There are thousands of variations on this theme. As a doctor, I have observed them in their many forms.

As you can't enjoy life and be frightened at the same time, it becomes necessary for you to take occasional inventory of yourself.

How much of a hypochondriac are you? Are you a Grade A, just normally apprehensive? Or are you far down the scale, a Grade Z, who worries about everything?

Whatever your designation I hold out better hope for you. Some kind of hypochondriac you will always be.

Therefore, your job is to learn how to be a happy hypochondriac. One who eats in peace, sleeps in peace, works and plays contentedly.

It's Normal to Be Anxious

But keep remembering that a certain amount of anxiety is normal. Patients sometimes say, "These tranquilizers I have been taking help me. But I can't say that they have removed *all* of my anxiety."

I tell them I am not in favor of super-duper tranquilizers. Blockbusters! Any drug devised to resolve every anxiety that a person has might be doing him a disservice. To survive—as I have indicated, and it bears repetition— we need to be a little anxious.

Suppose you weren't anxious when you crossed the street? How many times do you think you could make it safely? Why is a mother so careful to test the temperature of her baby's bath? Because she is anxious not to scald her infant. Why is a speaker anxious when he rises before his audience? Because he is anxious to please.

If there were no anxiety in the world, pedestrians would be exterminated, baby would be scalded, and all speeches would be dull.

Anxiety is a "divine unrest." It is one of the greatest allies of that great force we all have deep within us: Self-Preservation. Unless you are at least a little anxious about yourself you will not be healthy or live long. I am not beating the tom-toms to transform you into a hypochondriac; all I am saying is that a little anxiety is a good thing.

It helps you make adjustments within yourself, with

your friends, with your family. If you are not anxious to please you become a boor. If you are not anxious to succeed you become a failure. In a roundabout way I have been saying: Don't be too ready to reach for the tranquilizer bottle with every twinge of mental discomfort. If your doctor thinks that a few pills will be beneficial, will lighten your overburdened emotional load, then take them without question. But never, on your own, decide to dose yourself with sedatives or tranquilizers. As long as you live you will be anxious. That is normal. And it doesn't make good sense to keep on taking tranquilizers for most of your life simply because you are not completely free from anxiety.

Be Thankful for Tranquilizers

But when "you gotta, you gotta." So many persons who need help refuse to take the necessary treatment—whether psychiatric or in the form of tranquilizers. ("I don't fancy taking dope!") In spite of the apparently widespread use of these drugs as temporary crutches to get people over a bumpy trip during their lifetime, too many refuse because they look down upon the chronic pill-swallower as they do on the chronic alcoholic. The moral view has beclouded the down-to-earth need for the medicine. To give you an example of how tranquilizers can help in apparently hopeless patients, consider this letter received from Mrs. X. in Illinois. Even if you never need tranquilizers as much as she did, never hesitate to take them when your doctor prescribes them.

"*Dear Dr. Steincrohn:* I have just read in your column the letter from the 29-year-old mother of three who is so tired and nervous she can't stand it any more. I know so well how she feels. I have been through it. I hope I can help her. Therefore, please print what I write, for there is a *crying* need for understanding in the field of mental health.

"No one (except a psychiatrist) would have guessed that I was a neurotic. I was a model child, a good student, a calm bride, a serene mother. 'Easygoing' was the way I was always described. Never got angry, never lost my temper, never hated anyone, never blamed anyone, never got jittery.

Always Tired

"But then I began to get more tired than usual. I was so tired that I felt that I was barely existing. (I couldn't call it living.) And every few months I would (unknowingly) precipitate a falling-out with my husband, cry buckets of tears, and feel better till time for the next round.

"Although I had been tired most of my life, it got worse with each pregnancy and new baby. Doctors kept assuring me that there was nothing wrong with me. But soon I received a real shock to my nervous system. Seeing my mother die of a heart attack within one year, when she had apparently never had any trouble before, was more than I could stand. I was alone with her and the two young babies and couldn't get a doctor in time.

"Two months later, I was so nervous I often felt like screaming for no apparent reason. So I went to a doctor. (I had been very composed, by the way, at my mother's funeral.) This time my trouble was recognized as 'nerves,' and I was put on tranquilizers, much to my horror. I didn't believe in taking pills. But the results were extraordinary! I actually felt able to do my housework and be a good wife and mother.

"After two or three months on tranquilizers—I think I would have been dead without them—I still complained of extreme fatigue. My doctor referred me for psychiatric help. Not being able to afford a psychiatrist, I went to a Mental Health Clinic. I began feeling better immediately —just from knowing that something was being done for my tiredness; just to have someone realize that I really needed help; that I wasn't just lazy.

"My husband had always been most understanding and helpful, but my family felt that I was spoiled and lazy and that if I had only put 'mind over matter' I needn't have been tired. Imagination, they said! Even after I had been accepted by the Clinic, my brother was sure that if I just hired a baby sitter, got help with the housework, or took a part-time job to spark my interest in life and get me away from the daily grind—I would be all right. I know my brother had my best interests at heart and was deeply concerned about me. It was just that he was allergic to the word 'tranquilizers' and honestly mistrusted anything to do with psychiatry. And he is a highly intelligent, well-read man—but as you can see, misguided in his beliefs.

Take Mental Illness Seriously

"May I digress for a moment and say that his unwillingness to accept the idea that we humans have a mind that can get sick just as our body does, *and that we can't cure our mental ills by sheer will power*—this is what now makes me seethe with anger and with a desire to do something to dispel this stubborn ignorance, so that people will stop having to suffer as I have. And I realize that so many have suffered far more than I. (Please do not accuse me of self-pity.)

"The doctors I went to must have known about mental illness, yet until the last one, not *one* took me seriously enough to investigate the possibility that my trouble was nerves! And I still feel that my relatives don't really believe that I am emotionally ill.

"To get back to my story, I have now been going to the Clinic for a little over two and one-half years, and I feel I am nearing the end of my treatment and can look upon success in the offing. I couldn't possibly put into words how much the Clinic has helped. I am actually beginning to *live*.

"Perhaps your readers will be interested in what caused my neurosis. It would take too long if I went into detail. But in general, my exhaustion was caused by buried emotions. I used so much energy denying that I felt anger, grief (I couldn't even cry when my mother died, though I have always been quick to tears over trifles), that I had no energy left for living. I got plenty of sleep but little rest; because of dreams, nightmares, which I discovered, were the result of those buried emotions.

Repressed Feelings

"Let me hasten to explain that I had *no idea* I was burying my feelings. I had always been a communicative person. But it seems that the feelings that really mattered—those were the ones that I learned to deny so long that I have no recollection of so learning. I was simply brought up to 'be brave,' 'don't stoop to anger,' etc. I don't mean that we showed no emotion. I saw my father cry many times. Affection was openly displayed. My father kissed my brother when he went off to war. No pat on the back stuff for him. But some emotions, notably anger, hate, and fear, were understood to be taboo.

"But that's past history. I now have three boys (about 18 months apart) and I get more work done than I did before I had any!

"Please tell your readers, Dr. Steincrohn, not to raise their noses at tranquilizers, and not to refuse to take them —any less than if their doctor prescribed aspirin or bicarb tablets. I think they kept my head above water until such time as other doctors were able to really bring me out of danger.

"There is so much anxiety around. Let's wake up the nation some more on the subject of mental health."

Don't Be Afraid to Take Tranquilizers

"Tranquilizer" has become a household word. And like anything else, familiarity has induced contempt, largely unwarranted.

For example, consider two such tranquilizers: chlorpromazine and reserpine which came into use about a dozen years ago. They have become an invaluable aid in the management of patients who have mental disease. Referring to their importance, Allen E. Hussar, M.D., of Montrose, N.Y., reported in the *Journal of the American Medical Association:* "The practice of psychiatry changed and so did the internal order of the psychiatric hospital. Most of the locked doors opened; physical restraint disappeared; and insulin shock therapy became a thing of the past. Electric convulsive therapy remained in use, though on a much smaller scale, and need for wet-packs became exceptional." Without a doubt tranquilizers have become welcome additions in the physician's fight against anxiety and other mental problems.

Lately, however, I have noted that many think of tranquilizers as being an overrated fad. Perhaps overused when not really indicated, but certainly not overrated when definitely needed.

If your doctor believes that some kind of tranquilizer, of which there are many on the market, is indicated in your case, don't discard his advice because you have gotten the idea over some back fence that tranquilizers are already "old hat."

One of the reasons that some people won't take tranquilizers is because they have heard that they may cause skin rashes and other uncomfortable reactions. If that should happen, remember there is usually time enough for the alert doctor—if you see him in time—to discontinue the medicine. But remember that this is not a common occurrence limited only to the use of tranquilizers.

Drug Sensitivity

What we should not overlook is that any drug may cause an eruption. Somewhere there is a sensitive patient who just can't take it. Think of the millions of people who take aspirin for years without any trouble, yet there are those comparatively few who will bleed or get other severe reactions after one or two such pills.

Millions take penicillin without reactions, yet there is the minority who break out all over, and in some cases, even endanger their lives by taking it.

These are only two examples. Any apparently harmless drug is liable to cause skin reactions, anywhere from simple itching to severe blotches, blemishes or ulcerations.

If you are sensitive to certain hormones you can get a reaction from eating capons which were fed these hormones; from penicillin in milk; from preservatives or additives found in various kinds of food, medicines and drink.

Common trouble makers in addition to those I have mentioned are sulfonamids, phenophthalein, barbiturates and drugs which are commonly used to lower temperature (antipyretics). You may get skin reactions from gold treatments in arthritis, from griseofulvin in treating fungus, from practically any drug you can name that you take for a headache, laxative, tonic or other remedy known to most households.

Remembering all this, you will not refuse to take tranquilizers if your doctor prescribes them for anxiety or any other reason. Don't rely on your own judgments; have faith in your doctor.

Don't Surrender to Anxiety

When your doctor says "stop worrying" (thou shalt not have anxiety) he asks you to do the impossible. Perhaps we can learn to worry less but we can't stop. Just keeping alive is a struggle.

H. S. Burr, Emeritus Professor of Anatomy at Yale School of Medicine, wrote an interesting article on anxiety in *Connecticut Medicine*. He says: "In spite of the hundreds of years that man has lived, we really have gotten nowhere. We are troubled, we are frustrated, we are anxious, we have no adequate guide as to how to attack this problem or how to hope for a successful solution to it. Needless to say, there is no easy answer to this question; no single key that will unlock the riddle, nor is there any pink pill that will automatically guarantee a successful answer."

Nevertheless, we must keep trying. People can be taught to bear their anxieties either with the development of a new philosophy or with the help of tranquilizers until they are strong enough to match anxiety step by step. People who surrender to anxiety sink like a stone; others who fight to keep afloat make it to safety when all hope seems lost.

It is surprising to me why some doctors will actually

withhold sedatives or tranquilizers from patients who are anxious and afraid. They say, "I'm not prescribing medicine for your nerves. I want you to fight it out for yourself." And without further advice, the frustrated patients are left high and dry. Often, using the same line of reasoning, a physician will not give his patient a prescription for a few sleeping pills, although often a few good nights' sleep is the difference between recovery and a serious breakdown. Why this intrinsic aversion to offering the aid of temporary crutches? I could never understand it. On asking such physicians I would get vague answers: the chance of habit-formation, or reasons like "it's better to fight it out alone."

How Champions Overcome Anxiety

Anxiety being such a universal problem I became interested in how people who face imminent danger overcome their fears. What better than to interview a boxing champion in training for the defense of his title?

I interviewed Floyd Patterson in his training quarters about a week before his third fight with Johannson. Before the interview, I knew I would see what I saw: a superb physical specimen with rippling muscles beating like a machine-gun, rat-tat-tat; the final smash at the small bag that sounded like a clap of thunder. I saw him skip rope with the grace of a ballet dancer; and knock four sparring partners around in the ring as if they were stubborn puppets.

At last I got to the champion. I wanted to ask him how he overcomes fear and anxiety. There must be two parts to training for a fight: the physical and the emotional.

I wanted a simple formula for overcoming fear and anxiety that might help thousands of others; something for people who get up in mild anxiety and for those so frightened that they pull up the covers and cover their heads every night in fear.

I asked Patterson (a gentle man—and you make no mistake combining these two words into one), "How can a human being go into physical training for so many weeks before a fight as important as this one, without falling apart emotionally? What keeps you together at the seams? What prevents you from running out—in spite of the appetizing multimillion dollar gate? Isn't fear a greater force than love of money or power?"

He looked at me in that quiet way he has. Although he had just completed a jarring four rounds of boxing and work on the heavy and light bags, he sat there as if he were a reflective old man in a rocking chair. He emanated serenity and confidence. So kings must have sat on their thrones.

He was a good listener. I continued. I put it bluntly: "How do you train to overcome anxiety? Especially after the memory of that knockout in your first fight with Johansson? What do you do to wipe out the little devils who must be trying to stick little spears of fear into your mind? Can you sleep? Can you eat? Perhaps you can give me your secret. Think before you speak. For what you say may be a tremendous help to so many people who suffer from chronic anxiety, to many who have so lost faith that it seems they will never be able to hold up their heads and live their lives without the nagging fears that overwhelm them."

Simply and honestly he said, "I have no room for fear. I do not think of it; not that I am trying to run away from it. And I am not trying to build up my confidence by talking this way; it is a part of me. My days and nights are taken up with preparing my body so that it will be in top physical condition on the day of the fight. I think only of winning; never of the possibility of losing.

"I do my job, live day by day, and have faith. I guess you can call it positive thinking as much as anything else. I don't allow myself to think negative. If you want the secret that may help your patients perhaps it's in that last line: **Don't think negative.**"

On my way out of the hotel, I met another softspoken and renowned gentleman: former heavyweight champion Joe Louis.

I wanted to check and double-check on Patterson's formula. I asked him: "How did you train for a fight? Not your muscles, but your mind—so you wouldn't be scared?"

Like Patterson, he thought for a moment, and then said simply, "I was so busy with getting myself ready, there was no time for fear. I was always confident—not in any boastful way—that I would win. My manager used to say to me, just fight one round at a time, Joe. Then the next one, and the one after that. Until I won.

"In that way there's not time for fear. One thing at a time. People who think too far ahead can get themselves into a tizzy."

"That's the secret," Joe continued. "When you think only of winning, nothing can scare you. Too many people think of losing—and that makes them scared of life." (Could any psychiatrist have put it better?)

Don't Live Scared

So there you have it from two champions—one looking forward, the other back on the days of glory. Each with the identical formula for meeting life bravely. Live life one day at a time—courageously!

If you live scared, it's time you at least began to work hard at always thinking of winning. It's not easy but it's worth the effort. It works for champions, during the fearsome, awesome weeks of training. Why not for you against the small and large anxieties that bedevil every human being?

Stop worrying? Ridiculous. No human being can turn off worry like water in a faucet. But many things can reduce it to a trickle. Courage. Positive thinking. Tranquilizers (under a doctor's care). And the good sense to realize that it's silly to worry our lives away when there is so much we can do to neutralize anxiety.

Summary: Chapter 6

1. There are two large groups of nervous people. Those apparently healthy and those apparently sick.
2. People often withhold their anxieties from the doctor. They should tell all.
3. We live in an age of anxiety.
4. There is a difference between fear and anxiety.
5. Anxiety often begins after 35.
6. Don't be a Grade Z hypochondriac.
7. Weather can affect people with anxiety.

8. It's impossible to stop worrying altogether.

9. Menopause is a common cause of anxiety.

10. A person's reaction to an unfavorable environment often is a test for chronic anxiety.

11. Perhaps anxiety begins way back during the birth process.

12. We are all hypochondriacs in varying degrees.

13. Be thankful for tranquilizers. Don't refuse to take them if your doctor recommends them.

14. A case history of a patient with chronic anxiety. Re-read it to understand better how some people refuse to surrender to anxiety.

15. People aren't more sensitive to tranquilizers than they are to many other drugs.

16. There is a good lesson for us in how champions overcome anxiety.

The SIXTH Commandment: Thou Shalt Not Have Anxiety

Forget it IF:

1. You recognize that no-body is entirely free from anxiety.
2. You take tranquilizers without fear.
3. You believe that we shouldn't surrender to anxiety.
4. You know the difference between a Grade A and and a Grade Z hypochon-driac.
5. You realize that appre-hensive people often live longer.

Remember it IF:

1. You are always anxious.
2. You don't enjoy life be-cause of your apprehen-sion.
3. You have heard that tranquilizers are bad for you—and refuse to take them in spite of your doc-tor's orders.
4. You are in actual despair and deep in fear.

NOTE:

The understanding human being looks upon those afflicted with anxiety as those who need sympathy rather than derision.

NOTE:

Most persons with chronic anxiety live without hope of ever feeling better. Yet ex-perience shows that those improve who have the will to fight for weeks, months and —if necessary—for years against this stubborn enemy of mankind.

7

Thou shalt not
Be Under
Too Great Stress?

Through relaxation, you can meet life's challenges and become a truly happy person.

Anything that strains the human body is stress. Even the beating of the normal heart is stressful. I won't go into the part played by such glands as the pituitary or adrenals. All you need to know is that excess physical or emotional pressures can produce abnormal stress.

Stress Has Many Faces

For example, one man's pulse races and mouth dries whenever his alarm-clock goes off in the morning. He dislikes his job and he reacts stressfully.

A secretary's stomach knots up whenever her demanding employer asks her to work overtime on a batch of letters he has put off until the last moment.

Or, a middle-aged man, soft and flabby, decides to shovel a ton of snow off his sidewalk, and collapses with a coronary attack.

Stress is where you find it, and most of us find it in places that are specific for us alone. Nevertheless, we all react predictably in many situations. For example, investigators have studied the cholesterol levels of students taking exams. Practically all of them had higher readings after the tests. The cause? Stress produced emotions running amuck: fear, anxiety, intense concentration, etc.

Every thinking person will admit that tension is killing. It's not a by-product, but a product of modern life.

Tension can kill a coronary patient quickly—and an ulcer patient slowly. And we mustn't forget that the coronary and ulcer patients often got that way in the first place through tension.

A patient said, "I know I'm trying to crowd too much into 24 hours. If the day was only a few hours longer, I'd be less rushed."

I asked, "Suppose the good Lord had made the day 48 hours long. Do you think that would make any difference?"

He was in deep thought for a moment, then unwrinkled his forehead and smiled. He said, "No, I guess not. Probably would be twice as bad because it was twice as long. I'd just have more time to worry, hurry and scurry around."

Follow Your Doctor: Learn How Not to Live

One of the answers seems to be that it is not how much time we have but how we plan our day. A good way to learn how to live without tension is to follow the doctor around for 24 hours. (He's the one who tells you how to do it but—poor fellow—can't get around to regulating his own life.)

For example, consider how the doctor works, eats, sleeps and plays. The fight for a 30-hour-week amuses this man who is on call 168 hours weekly. He tells his patient: "Be sure to take at least an hour and a half for lunch"—but he himself takes a bottle of warm milk and a stale cheese sandwich at his desk.

He plans a vacation but cancels it because one patient is having a baby and another is having a hemorrhage. Tired, he looks forward to an eight-hour sleep and settles for four hours because an emergency gets him out of bed at three A.M.

The alarm clock bedevils him on other mornings and the telephone bell has him "hearing bells" all day. Now, all this is tension with a big T.

However, somehow doctors learn to take it. Otherwise most of us would be shuffled off at about 40. The answer seems to be a philosophical acceptance of the job and love for the work.

Once one of my colleagues said, "The only thing that keeps me happy and on the job is the realization that I'm helping human beings. If I had to work as hard as this for just dollars I'd give it all up today—even if it meant losing a million."

Do You Like Your Job?

In other words, it's the question of the square peg in the round hole all over again. If you like your job there is less chance you will be tense. It's easy to blame our tensions on the 20th century—and not on ourselves. A man comes in nervous and distraught. You ask him what's on his mind. His reply often falls within this pattern: "I work too hard. I try to do too much. I guess my job's getting me down."

Then you ask him how he likes his work. If he is honest and frank about it he will answer: "You may as well know what I haven't told a soul. Not even my wife. I hate my job. Just the thought of it tires me. I hate getting up in the morning because I'll soon be confronted with the day's drudgery. I hate going to sleep at night because I have nightmares about my job. I dislike it so. At 10 A.M. I'm already daydreaming about how nice it will feel getting through the day's work at five."

Is there any wonder that such men are tense and nervous? That daily, unremitting stress at last gives them high blood pressure, an ulcer or a coronary attack? I am often amazed that they last as long as they do.

In advising them, I tell them to face up to their problem. Otherwise, I say, it will slowly but surely squeeze the life out of them.

There are three main reasons why people may dislike their work. 1. They are unsuited for it by temperament. (For example, many a doctor I know would be happier as a lawyer or engineer, and vice versa.) 2. They are unhappy because they think they are being underpaid or unappreciated. 3. Their environment is an unhappy one. Working conditions are poor. Drafts. Bad lighting. Too little privacy. Bosses too strict. Uncongenial workers.

The answer to this kind of tension seems obvious. If finances and other conditions allow, better get out of there before an ulcer, or worse, does you in. In fact, consider it even if resigning causes financial hardships.

It is true that many men live under great stress for the opposite reason: they become obsessed with their work; they are the ones who "are in love with their job."

He Could Not Relax

I recall an incident during a vacation in Florida a few years ago. A man took the chair next to mine. Absorbed in an interesting book, I hadn't realized I had been there for quite a while.

The man said something like this: "I couldn't help observing you this morning, doctor. My guess is that you have been sitting here for at least three hours. How do you do it? I'd certainly like to know the secret. I'd give anything to be able to relax like you."

I recall saying at the time that some people are fortunate; by nature they know how to relax. Like the cat in the sun, they just naturally take to ease and restfulness. I added that such persons, unfortunately, are not in the majority. Most of us are tense and forever on the go. We must be doing things; otherwise we feel frustrated and unhappy.

Later this man's wife told me about him. Year after year he had vowed that his next vacation would be a restful one. Nevertheless, at the end of two weeks, he was a physical and mental wreck. He couldn't sit; he couldn't stand still; he couldn't loll in bed in the morning; he couldn't take an afternoon nap.

The result? They'd cut short their vacation and be back north weeks before they had planned to do so. But back in the busy routine of work, her husband felt like the fish that has been unhooked and thrown back into the water. He was again in his element—happy and fulfilled.

Many patients have asked me for a formula that will guarantee relaxation and freedom from stress and tension. I have told them that the fundamental requirement is the development of a new philosophy; that if stress can't be entirely prevented in normal living we can at least take sensible measures to neutralize it. For example, consider a common antidote against stress: vacations.

Need for Vacations

You can take a lesson from your heart on how to take vacations. It is very jealous of its rest periods. It doesn't contract a dozen times and then take a rest. It wouldn't think of working all day and putting off the well-earned rest until nightfall. The heart knows better. It rests after every beat.

In fact, the heart rests longer than it contracts. For example, systole (contraction) of the ventricle takes three-tenths of a second. Diastole (refilling) of the ventricle takes five-tenths of a second. The entire heart is quiescent for about four-tenths of a second.

Over the years I have heard hundreds of people say, "Me take a vacation? I don't need one. I haven't taken one in years." And when you try to explain that a vacation is a necessity rather than a luxury they insist, "It may be so for the other fellow. I happen not to need one to keep fit."

"Is it sour grapes or do you really feel that way about it?" I have asked. A few have really believed that vacations are unnecessary. But most have admitted that there are other reasons for their apparent disinterest. Like: "I can't afford to get away." "I'm afraid my business may be chewed to bits by competitors while I'm away." "It's so long since I've had one I don't think I'd know how to enjoy it."

When you are dealing with a convalescent, it is easy to convince him that a vacation is necessary for his recovery. You tell him to make reservations for a trip to Florida or Arizona. Within a few hours he will be calling you to say "everything's all set," or actually be waving the tickets under your nose to show how cooperative he is. Sickness has a way of helping the doctor get his point across.

Severe Illness a Good Teacher

It is with the supposedly rugged and healthy individuals that we have our major tussles. Also with those who **think** they are healthy because they feel well—yet show evidence of serious chronic disease.

For example, I recall a busy trial lawyer whom I was treating for duodenal ulcer. Like many an ulcer sufferer he would come down with exacerbations in the spring. The only treatment that would give him relief was absolute rest in the hospital for a few weeks.

Around February or March of each year, I used to say, "You've been through another back-bending year of work and stress. Why don't you plan to get away for at least a few weeks in April? It may forestall all the recurring trouble you get in the spring. It seems more sensible to spend a few weeks away on vacation than as a patient in a hospital."

His answers each year invariably followed this pattern, "Wish I could. Too busy. Besides, I haven't had a vacation in 15 years. I'm too much in love with my job."

I told him that his love for his work wasn't the reason for his job-tenacity. The real reason was an unconscious conviction that he was irreplaceable. He thought that the world couldn't get along without him. Or, to put it frankly, he was really afraid of losing clients to his colleagues.

One spring, this 45-year-old man had a massive hemorrhage. He was what we call "one of the lucky ones." We doctors thought he might not even last until we got him to the hospital for blood transfusions. But he did. He was in the hospital about six weeks. He was now so weak that he was no longer a formidable opponent: it was easy to convince him that he needed a vacation.

After that vacation experience, he has become the most "vacation-minded" person I know. He refuses to take work home weekends. He takes an extended winter and summer vacation. He and his wife will go off somewhere for a few days at the drop of a hat.

He has not had any recurrence of his ulcer trouble in many years. Recently he said to me, "The trouble with you doctors is that you **tell** patients to take a vacation; what you should do is **make** them. I'm almost thankful for that ulcer flare-up and hemorrhage that almost killed me. Otherwise, I might have remained stupid and lived out my life on a treadmill."

There's many an arm the doctor wishes he could twist; but all we can do is advise. My opinion is that any man or woman who lives his life without periodic rest and vacation periods to recharge is in imbalance. A friend asked Justice Brandeis why he took one-month vacations. He said, "I can do a year's work in 11 months, but not in 12 months."

Stress Is with Us Always

Stress is a natural component of existence. The mother undergoes stress in giving birth; the infant itself undergoes stress in the process of being born. For then on life is a matter of meeting the stresses of today so we can wake up to meet the stresses of tomorrow. In kindergarten, in grade school, in high school, in college, in business, in managing the home, in meeting the changes in adolescence and of middle age, in adapting to the apparent futility of aging—each one of us is bound to be burdened with stress and tension and anxiety. Our success or failure in meeting such strains will depend on how well we develop a practical working philosophy which can do the job.

For example, consider over-ambition. This might be called a bad-good habit. But it deserves a more specific terminology: obsession. It is natural to want to succeed, but unnatural to think success is so important that nothing else matters. You can see, if you will look around you, many examples of successful failures in your neighborhood and community.

Observe how, in passing, they have littered the road

with unhappy wives and children, with enemies who hate the ground they walk on, with "yes" men who respect them less than they realize.

Ambition, in normal amounts, is essential fodder for the ego. Man either *is* or *isn't*. He *is* when he moves—especially toward a higher goal. He *isn't* when he stagnates, when he allows potential greatness in himself to die of inanition and lack of desire for self-improvement.

Somewhere between the beachcomber (whose ego is close to zero on the social scale) and the driven man (who sits atop the heap) is the normal desire to make good. I would be the last to suggest that you give up your ambitions, but the first to remind you to realize your limitations.

Step Back and Look at Yourself

See yourself "in whole," not "in part." It is necessary that a man know where he wants to go; then assess his probabilities for arriving. Having these answers, he must also ask himself *how* he expects to achieve his ambition, and *when*. We can make mistakes all along the line; and these add up to various amounts of stress.

Some men work hard without knowing their destination, and not caring. Others, knowing what they want, over-assess their capabilities. Again, others know their destination and fairly estimate their innate capabilities, yet become successful failures because they have underestimated the time it takes to succeed. They burn themselves out prematurely. I call them "the impatient ones." Often, within reach of their goal, they turn off in another direction and fail.

To me, the extremely ambitious person who is unsuited for his calling is the saddest of all. To work all one's life thinking you are going in one direction and to find that you have only been marking time, or, worse still, have been going in an opposite direction: that is tragedy.

Intense ambition that is doomed to wreckage on the rocks because of inherent weakness in the ship is an awful thing to watch.

But suppose you are fit for your work. Your destination is well-lit. You see it clearly. You know your itinerary and how to use it.

Nevertheless, you may fail because you are not content to cruise slowly. You are the impatient man. You are bedeviled into taking short cuts, untried detours that wind you up into a maze of tension, doubt, indecision and final defeat.

Or, you too quickly reach your goal. You gather in much money, acquire power and respected stature in your community. When you do, balance your success against the price you have had to pay in loss of health, friends, and the happiness and companionship of your family.

Successful as you are, would you pay the price again? If not, there may still be time to recapture what you have lost on the way up.

Many Don't Realize They Are Tense

One of the obstacles you must overcome is being unaware that you are under great daily stress and tension.

You see, most people are tense without knowing it. They are unaware that they are wound up like a corkscrew.

For instance, many a wife has told me in the presence of her husband, "I can't understand what's come over Jim lately. He's so tense and touchy I can't say a word without him jumping down my throat. I wish you'd give him something for it, doctor."

I'd observe Jim as his wife spoke and disbelief would be written all over his face.

"Me tense?" he would say. "Why, Mary doesn't know what she's saying."

Without realizing it, he would be sitting up stiff and upright and his fists would be clenched in tension. Likewise, many a tense wife accused by her husband of being "snappy," acts just as surprised.

You cannot hit a target unless you know where it is. The more clearly you see it the more likely a bull's-eye. It must be evident, therefore, that you must take a good, long, unbiased look at yourself. If members of your own family tell you that you have been "difficult" lately, take heed. If your associates at the office or shop have dropped hints that you are not the same, sweet-tempered person you picture yourself to be, that should clinch it. If you admit it, you will be well on the way to overcoming your tension.

Don't Rationalize

Listen to Mr. S., businessman and philanthropist, who said recently:

"I, of all people, should have known that charity begins at home, but I had to learn the hard way.

"Isn't it funny how a person can rationalize away his bad qualities? For months I have been a rotten apple in the barrel of a sweet family. Before long I had my wife and four children upset and fearful every night when I returned from work. As for the long week-ends, they must have suffered the tortures of hell with me around. I was irritable, picked on everybody for no conceivable reason and was a bitter pill in more ways than one.

"But did I think I was tense and nervous? Not I! *Everybody else was unreasonable and hard to get along with,* I thought. It couldn't be sweet little me! And if I was occasionally a little edgy, didn't they all realize that I was tired and exhausted from working all day to give them roof and bread—and giving of many of my evenings to promote my charities?

"Doctor Steincrohn, not until my wife got sick—and almost died—did I at last wake up to the realization that I had been unreasonable and hard to live with. You'd be surprised how easy it is to get into the *habit of being tense.* It wasn't long after my wife got well, that we were a happy family again. And that was only because I at last admitted that I was living in tension and took steps to overcome it."

To remove tension you must not only recognize it, but remove the cause. Most often that is a job for your physician. First he must rule out possible organic disease (for example: unsuspected ulcer, hypertension, thyroid disease, heart disease, change-of-life, etc.). Not finding these, he will outline a new **way of life** for you. Before he can successfully accomplish this, he will have to spend much time with you, learning about your habits, your business and home life.

Definition

Dr. Hans Selye in defining *stress* in a talk a few years ago said, among other things, "What is stress? Anything that is too much is stress. It is impossible to live without stress."

Stress is where you find it:

You work under or with someone at the office whom you resent or dislike. That is stress.

You and your wife argue and shout. What were occasional skirmishes have turned into a daily battle. That is stress.

You come home from a hard day at the office to a sick and invalided child. That is stress.

Your wife is a hopeless cripple. That is stress.

You have mounting financial problems. That is stress.

You are an alcoholic. You are a chain-smoker. That is stress.

Return to the definition: "Anything that is too much is stress" and you soon realize that some form of stress is our daily heritage. **Thou Shalt Not Be Under Too Great Stress?** This is an enviable commandment but impossible to carry out. Days of great stress and tension are our lot in life. How to prevent stress from mounting and overcoming us, how to blunt its attacks which come in various guises: this is man's challenge.

Begin at the beginning. Prune your philosophical tree. Stand off and get a clear picture of your **way of life.** This is the basic foundation of the fight against stress and tension. There are questions you must ask and questions you must answer.

Answer These Questions

Are you happy in your work? Do you like your job, just accept it in boredom, or actually hate it? Do you overwork? Do you underwork? (Just work hard enough to collect your pay check?) Do you live in indecision? Are you envious or resentful of your colleagues? Do you take out your frustrations on your wife and children? You cannot evade such questions and hope to live a less stressful life.

If you do not like your job, change it! Life is too short to waste it in days and years of unfulfillment. Are you actually overworking? Then cut down. I don't go along with the theory that "you can't kill yourself by overwork." Try to overcome indecision which, although apparently harmless, is a breeder of stress. Does resentment against one or more co-workers have you in a blue funk every working day? Then get at the real reason for the resentment. If it is plain jealousy, root it out before it actually poisons your system with chronic illness. Have you become a despot at home because of what you "suffer" at the office? Then look at yourself in the mirror and be courageous enough to say: "Here stands a coward and a buffoon."

Ask and answer these and similar questions and you will have taken more than one giant step towards a way of life which is in itself an antidote against unbearable stress. You will find that it helps you to adapt to life and its many vicissitudes. It will give you direction in life; you will know your goal and more easily reach it. Less likely will you be one of those unfortunates who lose themselves in their work to run away from life. Like Miss N., for example.

Story of a Sad Girl

She was an apparently intelligent secretary in her thirties. She held an important position with a high official in one of our large industrial concerns. She complained of always being tired.

"I have to push myself," she said. "I go to sleep tired— and get up tired. I know the reason. My job's always on my mind. I even take work home with me every night."

She appeared a healthy specimen, and examination confirmed it. Her basal metabolism and protein-bound iodine tests revealed no thyroid trouble. She had no secondary anemia. She certainly did not suffer from lack of vitamins because she was well nourished and ate a varied and well-balanced diet.

In her case, the cause of her extreme tiredness undoubtedly was due to emotional tension and overwork. She was living in imbalance. She had few friends. She did not go to dances. She had no hobbies or other outside interests. Her family lived a thousand miles away, so she had actually cut herself off from all normal social contacts.

Yet, she seemed normal in other respects. She had a nice personality and was pretty. I wondered about the real reason for her unnatural withdrawal from society. It was not until she was ready to leave that I had a clue.

I told her that she ought to play more and work less. I said that her ambition was misdirected, that she was a healthy girl, that her symptoms were due to emotional and physical exhaustion. She agreed that perhaps she was overdoing but didn't see how she could change her work habits.

Then I wrote a prescription and said, "Take these pills as directed. They will eliminate much of your fatigue, provided of course, that you let up on your unremitting work and relax more."

"Are they something for my blood?" she asked.

"No," I said. "Your blood's all right."

"Are they vitamins?"

"No. You don't need vitamins."

"Then what are they?" she insisted. "I like to know what I'm taking. I like to know the reason for everything."

Then I tried patiently to explain the action of the medicine. But it was impossible, because she would have had to be a doctor herself to completely understand. So I told her the medicine would help her only if she had complete faith in it.

I said, "When you take a plane or train do you cross-examine the pilot or engineer? Do you ask about every detail of the machine's mechanism? I'm sure you don't. You fly and ride and do hundreds of other things in life on faith alone. Why not just take this medicine on faith?"

She had an answer ready. "I do not believe in faith. I want to know everything about everything. Besides, I don't like medicine. I never take it anyway. Thanks for everything."

I was extremely sorry for this girl. Holding down a responsible job and intelligent in conversation, here was a person maladjusted to the life around her. Her work-compulsion was evidence of her imbalance. Unquestionably, her compulsion to know the minute reason for everything had driven away all of her friends. Work was her only surcease from the nagging troubles deep inside. This "successful" private secretary was really a failure. She was a receptacle for a cross-current of stresses and tensions. She really needed psychiatric advice which she refused.

Unnaturally hard work can kill you emotionally as well as physically. If you find that your "work is your life" and nothing else matters, better take a detached look at yourself. You and your family deserve some pleasure as you go along from day to day.

Some Valuable Tips

There are the big stresses and the little stresses. So far I have tried to alert you to the need for a new philosophy to overcome the larger ones. But the smaller ones add up to a lot of unhappiness, fatigue and unfulfillment, too. For example, if you are a businessman, the following tips will help:

1. If you start your day in a rush and end it in a rush, try this: get up at least a half-hour earlier in the morning; don't let the hands of the clock bedevil you; be aware of time and be miserly about spending it.

2. Don't allow "time-snatchers" to take advantage of you. The man who puts his hand in your pocket and comes up with precious minutes robs you of more than if he came up with coin. Studiously avoid him; or let him know that you know that he is a time-thief.

3. Arrange an answering schedule for telephone calls. Don't return all calls immediately. Otherwise you will be

in constant tension between talking on the phone and consummating your work in the office. Set aside a time in the morning and the afternoon to bunch your answers.

4. Don't completely fill your appointment book. Allow time for unexpected interruptions.

5. Allow time for a leisurely lunch. What time you save by eating at your desk top you lose in energy.

6. Remember the value of naps. A couch in your office often will be a cheap premium as compared to a psychiatrist's couch.

7. Moderate exercise is often beneficial; overexercise is harmful.

8. Massage is a pleasant way to prevent and overcome tension.

Many a man finds happiness in his work but actually hates to come home to face the tensions which are piled up waiting for him as he comes through the front door. His wife can do much to take stress from the back of her man. The following suggestions are practical and have proved helpful to many patients:

1. Don't greet him with petty complaints as soon as he walks in: "Jimmy was called to the principal's office to be reprimanded"; "little Alice tore her new dress"; "the baby cried all day."

2. Give him a drink, let him stretch out with the evening paper and relax at least a half hour before serving dinner. Otherwise he will be too tired to eat or talk.

3. Be a good listener when he begins to get things off his chest.

4. Try to prepare yourself for the added home stresses when your husband returns from work and the kids come home from school. Learning to take a rest period and tak-

ing time to freshen up will take much tension out of the evening "togetherness."

Keep remembering that I have not been trying to show you how to eliminate stress entirely from your life. To live is to be stressful. I have only been trying to lighten the load. To make you aware that stress can be both normal and harmful. Stress in excess adds up to physical and emotional trouble. The individual who masters the art of living with as little stress as possible, is the happy person. Because stress is the Number One poison of modern existence.

One of the best tranquilizers I know is a dip into the thoughts of Marcus Aurelius Antoninus. In his sayings, comes forth the wisdom for living life as it should be lived. One of my favorites is this: "Do not act as if thou wert going to live ten thousand years. Death hangs over thee. While thou livest, while it is in thy power, be good."

Reread that a few times and shortly you will find that tension and stress fall away from you and leave you relaxed and thankful to be alive.

Chapter Summary

1. Nobody is free from stress or tension.
2. Follow your doctor around for 24 hours and learn how NOT to live.
3. Job hatred is a common cause of stress.
4. Vacations are useful antidotes against stress. However, not everyone knows how to relax.
5. Take a lesson from your heart on how to relax.

6. Many think that vacations are unnecessary—until they are struck down by serious illness.

7. You invite stress if you are over-ambitious.

8. Often we are tense and under great stress without realizing it. Only our family, friends and associates see it clearly.

9. To be able to lessen tension you must first be able to recognize it.

10. "Anything that is too much is stress." Both the office and the home are breeding grounds for abnormal tensions.

11. Stand off for a clear picture of yourself. Perhaps you need to develop a new philosophy: a new **way of life.**

12. Reread tips on how to lessen stress at work.

13. Reread tips on how the wife can save her husband.

The SEVENTH Commandment: Thou Shalt Not Be Under Too Great Stress

Forget it IF:

1. You have a good working philosophy of life.
2. You love your job.
3. You know how to relax.
4. You are not overly ambitious.
5. You like to come home because it is free from abnormal tensions.

Remember it IF:

1. You have no direction or destination.
2. You dislike your job.
3. You are quarrelsome and tense at home and at work.
4. You wonder how much longer you can keep on "carrying your heavy and unbearable load."

NOTE:

Some people are "born happy." But most of us have to *learn* to be happy and live with a minimum of stress. If your days are filled with stress and tensions find a new Way of Life. It is essential if you expect to get some fulfillment out of existence.

NOTE:

A safe and sure way to overcome the problem is to presume you are tense. As most people are, chances are that you are, too.

Therefore, practice at counteracting stress. Learn to "detensify." When you have learned your lessons well you will begin to live—for the first time.

8

Thou shalt not
Become a Victim
of Your Emotions?

Your thoughts can keep you healthy and happy.

In every branch of human activity you will find a few men who are proud to be called skeptics. Medicine also breeds such people who perversely think they grow in stature in proportion to the bigness of what they tear down. Nevertheless, many of these disagree with the majority opinion for no other reason than that they honestly question the accepted beliefs.

Psychosomatic Medicine

The other day a few doctors were discussing psychosomatic medicine. Every once in a while it has a way of popping up into medical shop-talk. All of us, but one, admitted that this concept of the patient and his ailments has advanced our medical understanding by hundreds of years.

And then the conversation got around to one of our colleagues who is intensely interested in this phase of practice. The unbeliever, a fine chap who questions the significance attached to mind over matter (and vice versa) said, "I think Dr. Z. is getting cracked in his ideas about psychosomatic medicine. First thing you know he'll be saying people can talk themselves into having cancer! After all, there's a limit."

I agree that people can become overenthusiastic. Yet, I think that the psychosomatic-minded doctor is the better practitioner of the two. There's less chance of selling the human being short if you consider him in his entirety. Likewise, there's less chance of helping him (both body and mind) if you look upon him only as a "heart" or "liver" or "kidney" case.

Although it has been repeated so many times that it is almost a cliche, it is nevertheless true that "it is just as important to know who has the disease as it is to know the disease he has."

In a paper appearing in the *Journal of the American Medical Association*, April 16, 1955, Dr. Francis J. Braceland, Psychiatrist-in-Chief of Hartford's Institute of Living, said in part: "Despite all criticism, psychosomatic medicine is an excellent method of approach to medical practice, for there can be no medical practice, including psychological medicine, that is not psychosomatic if it deals with people. The human being of necessity is a person who is constantly involved in psychological, biological, sociologic and economic processes and adjustments within the framework of his environment."

One of the essential requisites for being a good physician is that he has *large ears*. By that term I mean that he is sympathetic, understanding, kind and patient. Only by having such qualities, either inherent or acquired, can any doctor be of the greatest help to his patient.

If you have ever been troubled or ill you will understand what I mean. Either you have been blessed with such a physician or you have gone from one office to another in search of such a one.

Organ Language

I can only guess that such a sympathetic doctor was the late Dr. Edward Weiss, Professor of Clinical Medicine at Temple University. It was he who first suggested that many patients talk in "organ language."

Here are some examples of organ language:

A patient comes to the doctor complaining that he can't swallow. All the necessary diagnostic tests are negative. But the careful doctor goes into the patient's history and finds that there is something in the patient's life situation that "he can't swallow." For example, a tyrant-like, unappreciative boss at the office.

One man complains of nausea. The only cause is a distressing home problem that he "can't stomach."

A girl complains of "loss of appetite." The doctor discovers that she becomes physically starved because she is emotionally starved. She also has "fatigue" which is due to emotional conflict.

In another, a "neuralgia" is due to muscle tension

aused by emotional tension. In still another, an "ache
n the arm" may be caused by the fact that the patient
would like to strike someone but can't because of respect
mingled with hostility.

A patient may come in complaining of "itching." Sometimes this represents his dissatisfaction with his surround-
ings. So he scratches himself instead of someone else.

In the same manner, other symptoms are due to difficulties in his environment that the patient can't overcome.
Therefore, he gets anxiety feelings, shaky legs and what
he thinks are heart attacks.

I want to stress that every symptom you have cannot
be explained on a psychiatric or psychosomatic basis. That
would be foolhardy. Believing that, we would miss the
diagnosis of serious underlying organic disease. Our job
is first to use every diagnostic test indicated by a careful
physical examination to rule out organic disease. This
having been done, we should not make light of fears,
phobias and other complaints. For the emotions are powerful forces that make terrific impact on our physical selves.

Hyperventilation

As an example of a common condition that is often
overlooked, consider what we call hyperventilation. This
is a technical term for overbreathing. Although most of
us think of breathing as one of the most natural attributes
of our physical machine ("as easy as breathing"), thousands of persons, apparently healthy, suffer disquieting
symptoms caused by a breathing apparatus that has gone
out of whack.

Usually such people are nervous and tense. They do

not even suspect that they have been breathing abnormal
ly. Let me tell you how it works out.

For example, here is a 35-year-old office worker who
has been complaining of left chest pain and "difficulty
in breathing." Otherwise, he says, he has had no com
plaints except occasional giddiness and numbness of hand
and feet. As you observe him, you see that he is unsmiling
and edgy. He sits there taking abnormally deep breaths
as he talks to you. He has what we call a sighing respira
tion.

"No matter how deep I breathe," he says, "I can't
seem to get enough air. I don't have the satisfaction, like
I used to, of feeling my lungs full." He can't understand
what is wrong. He is worried about his heart because of
his chest discomfort. He is a typical cardiophobe.

Complete physical examination is negative. Chest x-
rays, electrocardiograms and blood studies give this man
a clean bill of physical health. Going deeper into his history, we learn that the symptoms began about six months
ago, when he failed to get the promotion he thought was
due him.

His wife noticed that he used to sit around and sigh
a lot. When she called it to his attention, he either denied
that he was sighing or said that he couldn't stop it. His
was unquestionably a case of hyperventilation.

Quite often, dramatic reproduction of his symptoms
will convince such a patient what is wrong. Just telling
him that his emotions are the cause is not enough.

I said, "I will prove to you what is causing your symptoms. I am going to ask you to breathe as deeply as you
can, as fast as you can, until I ask you to stop. After 30
or 40 deep breaths—making certain to expel as much air
as you can with each expiration—your hands and feet

ill begin to tingle and get numb. Your chest will feel eavy and you will get dizzy and feel faint."

After about 30 deep breaths he began to feel dizzy. Ie stopped before he felt worse. After a few minutes of reathing normally again, he said, "Doctor, that heavy reathing made me feel like you said it would. I can see here must be some connection between my sighing all he time and the way I have been feeling." I gave him sedative and told him how to try to control his deep reathing and sighing. His wife said she would keep call- ng his attention to it. After six weeks all of his symptoms lisappeared. He got out of the habit of sighing by accept- ng his job-setback and taking it like a man instead of mmaturely.

The Physiological Reason

Physiologically, here is what happens to cause such a patient's symptoms. When you breathe normally, you do not disturb the fine balance between oxygen and carbon dioxide in the blood. However, deep breathing causes an ncreased loss of carbon dioxide. The hemoglobin of the blood clings to oxygen more than usual. As a result, the body's tissues are deprived of oxygen. The brain, being very sensitive to oxygen loss, produces such symptoms as anxiety, dizziness, faintness, numbness of hands and feet. Patients with this condition (called alkalosis) also com- plain of being weak and tired. They have a fear of black- ing out. They may have difficulty in swallowing, have stomach cramps and a lump in the throat.

Of course, all nervous patients with hyperventilation are not so easily cured as the young man I have just told

you about. Many nervous persons have unconscious
been overbreathing for years. They meet every proble
and difficult situation with deep sighs, or with shallo
rapid breathing, which after a while causes alkalosis ar
the symptoms I have mentioned.

Cure requires patience on the part of the patient, wl
usually improves when his basic anxiety is overcome. Th
less he worries the less he overbreathes. If you have bee
distressed lately by similar symptoms, look to your breatl
ing. It may be hyperventilation.

The sick carry heavy loads. So do the healthy. There
fore, as fellow human beings, we should not inadvertent
add to our neighbors' discomforts. Emotions are easil
played upon. Often people become tactless without reali
ing it.

Tactless Grandmother

For instance, the other day I heard this incident. A
thirteen-year-old girl had recovered from a severe bou
with a strep throat. It was her first day out of bed. Sh
was peaked, wan and weak.

Her grandmother, who loved her very much, had come
for the day to help with the housework. At lunch time
grandmother, mother and daughter sat around the kitcher
table. The little girl was the topic of conversation.

"Don't you think Jane looks well?" inquired the mother.

"Looks well," answered Grandma, "I was just going to
say she looks like death itself. I never saw Jane look so
horrible. Are you sure the doctor can't do something
more for her?"

And she kept repeating this devastating talk throughout the day. After Grandmother left for her own home at the end of the day, Jane had a relapse. "She had to go back to bed for a few days. She was hysterical. You never saw such a scared child in your life."

If You Can't Say a Good Word—Say Nothing

We can be morale builders for our friends as easily as we can unduly cause them concern. Have you ever started out in the morning, fresh, vibrating with energy, and eager to work, only to run into some killjoys?

"You don't look well, Tom. What's the matter? Not feeling well?" You try to pass that off lightly, then you encounter the second one: "Tom, why don't you get away for a while? Never saw you looking so beat."

If you react like most humans, your early morning bounce will soon be dissipated. You will be examining yourself closely in the mirror. "Perhaps they are right," you will think.

A good rule is this: never tell a heart patient he looks bad—or anyone else, even if he does. You may make a sick person sicker, and a well person sick. Next to being told we are looking young, most of us like to be told we are looking well.

If we are ill we like to feel we are getting better. If we are well we dislike the thought of possible illness in the offing. The sick person deserves all the moral support he can muster. In some extreme cases, doctors think that an uplifting white lie is preferable to depressing silence in answer to the patient's question about his condition.

A good precept to live by is this: if you can't say a good word to a fellow being, better not say anything.

This attitude works out well whether the one you address is healthy or sick.

Anxiety—the Number One Problem

After a lecture I was asked if it wasn't true that anxiety is the number one problem of human existence. I agreed. Unquestionably we live on a stage whose backdrop is a black curtain of fear and anxiety. Whether the cause is preoccupation with H-bombs, hurricanes, health or financial insecurity, we human beings are besieged by daily uncertainties.

Only the truly philosophical, who are comparatively few, seem to be able to take life in stride. They live in tranquility and contentment. Many intensely religious people are in this group. The Bible and the way of life it prescribes, acts as a soothing balm on wounds of the spirit and body.

Another listener asked, "What else would you say is up there near the head of the list? What other things plague most people?"

I answered that resentment deserved a high place of dubious distinction. I have known hundreds of patients who might have been well had they been able to eliminate from their minds this poisonous emotional turmoil. I cited one case that stands out vividly. It shows how resentment can put a hole in your stomach.

Resentment and Ulcer

The patient was an executive in his late thirties. Previously healthy, he began to complain of stomach symptoms. Not responding to medication and diet, he entered the hospital for observation. X-rays showed a small duodenal ulcer. After months of specific treatment he did not improve. Subsequent x-rays showed that his ulcer was larger. (He had given up cigarettes, alcohol, and was a completely cooperative patient.)

Under questioning during all these months of treatment, our man continued to be his smiling, apparently happy, self. There were no complaints of excessive tension at home; everything was all right at the office.

One day he came in complaining of the increased severity of his pains. "I can't sleep. The pains wake me every morning at about two. Milk helps stop it, but by that time I'm unable to fall asleep again. My mind keeps going round and round."

I asked him what his revolving mind kept thinking. As usual he clammed up tight. He came in one week later. This time he talked. For the first time in months of treatment, he opened up the flood gates, and repressed hatred and resentment poured out.

"For months I've hated my closest friend. He doesn't even suspect it, because I've been outwardly as nice as ever. He's completely innocent but I haven't been able to forgive him for getting the promotion at the office which I feel I deserve. Every time I look at him, or even think of him, my stomach bunches up." (He clenched his fist to show me how much.)

Value of Ventilation

I told him that now, at least, we had some chance of curing him. While he continued to be resentful all the medicines and special diets we gave him were actually going down the drain. If he would follow through and find some way to get rid of his hatefulness, he would begin to feel better.

After much discussion he agreed to talk out his resentment with the man he hated. Confession is not only good for the soul; it is good for stubborn ulcers, too. It took courage, but he did it.

When he returned to the office a few months later the hollows in his cheeks had filled in. He looked a healthy specimen. "Do you know, doctor," he said, "it was the most difficult thing I ever had to do in my whole life. But almost like a miracle, after I spilled out my crazy resentment to him, it was as if an invisible hand removed a sharp, boring instrument from my stomach and coated the spot over with some balm. I seemed to get better immediately."

It wasn't his imagination. Within months x-ray evidence of his ulcer disappeared. He has been symptom-free for at least 15 years. Incidentally, for the past 10 years he and his friend have been partners in their own business. Resentment is a poison they never have to contend with.

An ulcer? High blood pressure? A coronary attack? Such are too high a price to pay for the questionable pleasure of hating somebody.

Many people take their emotional problems as a matter of course. On the one hand they take their medicines and follow the doctor's directions, but on the other— as if applying a handbrake against their progress to recovery—they fail to deal with the emotions that keep health at bay.

Experiment at Cornell

Resentment? Anxiety? Fear? Hate? Too many consider these as normal components of existence. They do not realize that chronic hate, envy or jealousy are actually poisons that bedevil the arteries and vital organs.

In an experiment at Cornell some years ago scientists were able to observe a man who had a permanent opening in his stomach due to an accident in childhood. They could actually see how the stomach wall reacted to induced fear, anxiety and resentment.

For example, when the experimenters said something to induce anger in this patient, they looked through the opening in the stomach and saw that the mucous membrane of the stomach had turned fiery red, and was covered with many small hemorrhages. The stomach contracted more rapidly than normal and there was a marked increase of secretion of hydrochloric acid.

All this was a direct response to anger. These changes usually cleared up within an hour or two, after the experimenters convinced the patient that there was really no basis for his anger and resentment. But consider how, as in the case of our friend with the ulcer, continued resentment for months takes it out on the stomach and other organs. Chronic resentment will aggravate diabetes and cause the patient to spill more sugar; it will aggravate the toxic thyroid patient; it even brings on attacks of asthma in the susceptible.

Now, I realize we are all human. Hostility is a potential in each one of us. We hate. We resent. We are not saints.

But it is the depth and duration of the hostility and resentment that do the dirty work on the human machine.

Admit Your Emotional Problems

Therefore, if it is evident that you are having emotional difficulties with others, it is essential that you admit
something needs repair. Aggression and resentment need
early neutralization or they get out of hand.

Whom do you dislike and why? Do you bottle it up
and secretly praise your moral strength in hiding your
real feelings? You may be building up your ego on a
mushy foundation, and inviting serious organic damage
to your body. Have the courage, again like our ulcer
friend, to talk it out. Explode if necessary. Unnatural
containment of the poison of resentment will inevitably
cause illness somewhere.

If you are by nature a "hater" be a good one. A
friendly, popular man I know says: "Everybody hates
at times. The secret is to be a good hater. I'm a good
one. I get over it quickly. I may hate for a minute or,
rarely, for an hour—but never for weeks or months. What
does it get you but misery?"

Consider how chronic resentment is often the cause
of anxiety, which is a poison in itself. I have seen it in
hundreds of patients who worry unnaturally about their
hearts. They become cardiophobes. If they have an innocuous heart skip they are sure that they will one day
drop dead suddenly. Although the doctor has made a
complete cardiac survey and has repeatedly assured them
that they have a normal heart, they persist in their belief
that their heart is weak. A palpitation spells finis. They

translate an ordinary muscle sprain on the left side of the chest into angina pectoris. It's hard to convince them that shortness of breath on climbing stairs is, in their case, due to excess weight rather than due to a bad heart.

Emotions Can Affect Any Organ

Emotions most commonly affect the heart, which has been accepted as the center of emotions for centuries. But no organ is excluded. See what fear does. It dries your mouth, dilates the pupils of your eyes, sets your heart pounding in your chest. Before taking an important examination you may get diarrhea or have frequent desire to urinate.

Such are but a few common, recognizable reactions to the strong power of emotions on our physical being. Is it any wonder then that worry, resentment, hate, fear, anxiety and other strong emotions may be the cause of chronic diarrhea caused by an underlying colitis? Is it any wonder that anxiety may cause a nervous cough, heart symptoms, stomach and intestinal symptoms, headaches, skin symptoms? Few organs are free from the powerful action of emotions.

Are You Neurotic?

Are you a neurotic? Few persons will answer "yes" even though they are more than suspicious. In fact, those who admit they are may consider themselves already on the way to improvement or cure. Like the chronic alcoholic—a neurotic will rarely improve unless he admits he is one, and is willing and has the desire to get better. Otherwise, visits to the doctor's office and hundreds of tranquilizer pills will be completely ineffectual.

Here is how you may be able to recognize what you haven't previously admitted, that you are a neurotic, and that your life is being influenced by abnormal emotions.

Chances are that you have a phobia. You have an unreasonable fear: like being afraid to ride in a train, auto or elevator. You can't get up enough courage to go to church or to a movie. When you do try, you make certain to sit in an aisle seat, so you can get up and run out of there when the sudden fear overtakes you. You are afraid to remain at home alone. You are afraid to pick up a knife to pare the potatoes when the children are in the kitchen because you have to overcome the desire to use the knife on them. You are afraid that you are going crazy or will soon die.

You will note the repetition of the word *fear*, a word which seems to be tied in with most neurotic reactions. But the recognition is much easier than our ability to tear it out by the roots. It is a stubborn plant. The patient often continues to suffer for months and years. He may have symptoms that seem unrelated to his neurosis, nevertheless they are a part of it. For example, overdrinking and oversmoking, chronic depression, impotence and other sexual problems.

Majority Can be Helped

A majority of patients can be cured, but it is a long process. The psychoneurotic requires patient treatment to rehabilitate him. It takes daily visits to the doctor or clinic for months or years. The patient's environment often needs to be changed or improved. Often members of the family and associates at business must cooperate if improvement is expected.

Thou shalt not become a victim of your emotions? Stop worrying? Such are the common admonitions we hear at home, at business and in the doctor's office. It is not as simple as that. Emotions need to be held within normal bounds. The doctor can help. The family can help. So can friends. But anyone who has been through the hell of chronic anxiety will tell you that, in the end, victory or defeat depends upon the courage and valor of the person himself. And they will add that no trial of courage exceeds that experienced in trying to gain victory over one's emotions.

Chapter Summary

1. Psychosomatic medicine is more than a fancy name.
2. The psychosomatic-minded doctor is the better practitioner.
3. "It is just as important to know who has the disease as it is to know the disease he has."
4. A good physician must have "large ears."
5. Various parts of the body speak an "organ language."
6. Review the effects of hyperventilation.
7. Tactfulness is especially important where health is concerned.
8. Resentment ranks next to anxiety as a health problem.
9. Resentment can bore a hole in your stomach, raise your blood pressure, disable your heart.

10. It is important to admit that you have emotional problems.
11. Anxiety causes many to suffer Imaginary Heart Trouble.
12. Are you a neurotic? The first step in overcoming distressful emotions is to admit that you need help.

The EIGHTH Commandment: Thou Shalt Not Become a Victim of Your Emotions

Forget it IF:

1. You can answer honestly that you are a happy, well-adjusted, well-motivated person.
2. You are content with your vocation.
3. You have many outside interests.
4. You have normal, happy relationships with your family members and friends.

———

NOTE:

Individuals who are apparently well-adjusted should not look upon neurotics with disdain.

Each of us, however strong, has a breaking-point if the pressures become too great.

Therefore be thankful for your present state of well-

Remember it IF:

1. You harbor abnormal hostility and live with a chip on your shoulder.
2. You resent both your friends and your enemies.
3. You are abnormally jealous and envious.
4. You are quick to anger and slow to cool off.
5. You are beset by fears and phobias.
6. You keep insisting your symptoms are due to organic disease in spite of your doctor's assurance to the contrary.
7. You are unquestionably neurotic.

———

NOTE:

Some of the unhappiest patients I have known—not barring those who have cancer or heart disease—are

The EIGHTH Commandment: Thou Shalt Not Become a Victim of your Emotions (Continued)

being, and never downgrade the power of emotions in causing illness.

the psychoneurotics. For them the act of living from day to day is an actual challenge.

Fortunately, perseverance and fortitude bring improvement and cure in the majority of such people.

9

Thou shalt not
Have Too Many Doctors?

You can develop a happy doctor-patient relationship that will ease your mind and protect your health.

Patients sometimes get peculiar ideas. I do not say this in derision. One can only be in sympathy with laymen when they get lost in a forest of symptoms, discomfort and anxiety. One of the ideas they have is this: when in doubt concerning one's health, one must make a trip out of town to receive real medical advice and treatment.

Fear of Cancer

For example, recently I saw a patient who had been to five doctors within a few weeks. He had been complaining of vague abdominal pain. His wife having died within the year of cancer, he had become alarmed about his condition. "Perhaps it's cancer," he thought.

Not satisfied with the recommendations of these doctors, each one an outstanding man in his respective specialty, he is now considering going to clinics in Massachusetts, New York or Minnesota for a "complete workup."

As he had come to me for advice, I did not consider it fair to dissuade him from seeking help at the diagnostic clinics he had in mind. I agreed that he was certain to have excellent doctors and a fine diagnostic workup at these places. However, I also felt it necessary, in rounding out the complete picture, to inform him that he was seeking in the distance what lay closely at hand.

Distance Lends Enchantment

In effect, here is what I told him:

"Many people have the erroneous idea that a specialist is a fellow that lives at least 100 miles out of town. In other words, the farther you have to travel to see him, the bigger the specialist he is.

"Now it happens that you have been examined by five doctors in your own city who have carefully investigated you inch by inch. They have found no evidence of cancer. Physical examination and X-ray evidence are entirely negative.

"Your trouble is that you are now suffering from cancerphobia. You translate every little ache or pain into cancer because you stood by so long seeing your wife suffer from cancer. My advice to you is to believe your local doctors who have found you free from cancer. Take a vacation for a few weeks to break up the tensions you have been under during the past year. If, on your return, you still feel like having a checkup in a clinic, better go ahead and get it off your mind."

He followed my advice and improved under the care of the local doctors. An important factor in his recovery was the development of a new love interest while on vacation. He had been a lonely and introspective man.

I am not suggesting that traveling to a distant clinic or doctor is always a waste of time and money. I have often made such recommendations myself. However, it is well to remember that distance lends enchantment where doctors are concerned. Your own doctor, if qualified to do the job, may be as good, or better, than the fellow you are planning to see hundreds of miles distant.

Think it over before you go about packing your suitcase. Go ahead if your doctor recommends it. But better not make such a decision on your own judgment. This holds true whether you have cancer fears, heart disease or any other ailment.

Years ago, in speaking of a friend's demise, a philosopher wrote: "He died of too many doctors."

Medical Merry-Go-Round

I have had the opportunity to observe actual cases where this was true. Too many impatient people have a tendency to jump on the medical merry-go-round. They are forever looking for the brass ring, the "perfect doctor." There "ain't no such animal" any more than there is the perfect wife or husband, the perfect lawyer or the perfect day.

When a new patient comes in, prefacing his recital of complaints with this statement: "You're the ninth doctor I've been to. None of the others seem to know what's wrong with me. They haven't helped."—I am certain that Doctor #10 will soon enter the picture.

Some patients are impatient by nature. Whatever their disease, they expect to be made more comfortable within a few days or weeks. It is manifestly impossible to overcome the effects of long-standing, chronic illness within days. For example, the stubborn headaches sometimes associated with hypertension may resist treatment for months. The nagging aches and pains of arthritis may recur day after day in spite of cortisone drugs and other treatments. The diabetic may continue to spill sugar and have trouble with his vision in spite of the best management. The angina patient continues to have his chest pains and the woman in menopause still has her hot flashes. Impatience is frequently found in persons who have fears and abound with symptoms for which no organic cause can be found.

There is actual danger in going from doctor to doctor without giving the first a fair chance. For example, many have died because they refused to accept bad news and preferred to believe the doctor (sometimes a quack) who promised an easier and cheaper cure.

Procrastination Is Deadly

For example, Mrs. H. comes in concerned about a lump in her breast. Her doctor suggests immediate surgery to determine if it is cancerous. He adds that there is a possibility that the breast may have to be removed.

Being human and subject to human anxiety, she goes to another doctor—and another. Each says the same thing. But she keeps trying some more, in the hope that she will find one who will say all these doctors are wrong. "Of course you haven't got cancer. You don't need an operation. I'll cure you with special medicines."

The medicine the last man prescribes (perhaps doctor number six or number eleven) is harmless but the loss of time is deadly. The cancer spreads and the patient dies—a victim of the medical merry-go-round.

Stubborn Ulcer Patient

Or, here is an ulcer sufferer. His disease is under control. His acute stomach pains have disappeared, his appetite is good and he feels very much better. However, he rebels at the restrictions in diet. He says life is not worth living without his cigarettes and an occasional highball. But his doctor insists that he toe the mark if he intends to keep his improvement.

But the patient is a stubborn cuss. He has heard that the best thing to do for duodenal ulcer is have an operation. He goes to another doctor who also insists that medical treatment has proved itself in his case, and that an operation is out of the question. After he has consulted his sixth or seventh physician he finds one who agrees that operation is worth the gamble.

At the hospital a greater part of the stomach is removed and our patient returns home. He finds that his digestion is worse than it has ever been, that a drink upsets him, and that cigarettes are distasteful. A new element enters: extreme fatigue. He can't keep up his former business pace, loses his executive position, and is soon a "nervous wreck." Psychiatric treatment is ineffectual. He struggles along for a few more months and commits suicide.

There are other reasons than impatience to cause patients to roam from their doctor and try someone else. Often your doctor is guiltless. If your doctor tried to be "all things to all men" he would soon be requiring psychiatric care. He can't possibly please everybody: should he be verbose when faced with a patient who likes a talkative doctor; should he become the silent sphinx with his next patient who doesn't react well to a doctor who is "always gabbing"?

The doctor's sanity depends upon a simple resolution: Doctor, Be Yourself! Those who will like you, will; and those who will not, won't. The whys and wherefores of patients' likes and dislikes are difficult to fathom.

Is Your Doctor an Alarmist?

Especially is this true when a fine physician unjustly has this label pinned upon him by his community: *alarmist!*

I have known a number of physicians who were never able to live down this unearned reputation. As a result, their practices were not as large as those of their more optimistic colleagues and the community suffered for not placing more confidence in them.

Admittedly, there are a few doctors who are so tactless in handling an anxious patient that they frighten him. There is no excuse for this. However, I have known many a tactful physician who got the "alarmist" label simply because he was a thorough man who was doing his best for his patient. I recall one excellent diagnostician who suggested an x-ray series to a man who had been having indigestion.

The patient asked, "What do I need pictures for?" The doctor said, "It's just a routine investigation to make sure everything is all right." And the patient came back with this: "Oh! So you're looking for trouble. I suppose you're one of those fellows who's always looking for cancer or something like that." The patient stalked out of the office muttering "alarmist" and never came back.

Be Thankful for Doctor's Thoroughness

I tell people to be thankful that their doctor is thorough. Often life depends upon it. He often has to make the choice between scaring you and letting you die. From personal experience, I can tell you that it's much easier to pat a patient on the back and tell him everything is O.K. without going through an expensive, or frightening, rigmarole of diagnosis. The good doctor will not fear the Alarmist label. He will do whatever is necessary to keep his patient healthy and alive. Naturally, he wants his patients to like him and have confidence in him. But he will not surrender his principles of good practice "just to be popular." In time, just as water seeks its own level, so does the public discover who are the good doctors.

For example, in writing of the need for early cancer detection, in the *New York State Journal of Medicine,* Dr. Charles S. Cameron noted: "With all due respect and credit to recent trends, the office instrument of greatest value in the diagnosis of early cancer is still a well-developed sense of suspicion. No doctor should fear the reputation of alarmist as much as he should fear the responsibility for an avoidable death."

Definition of Good Physician

Here is my definition of a good physician: *one who looks for the worst but hopes for the best*. Think carefully before discharging a doctor because you label him an alarmist. He, rather than doctor number seven or ten may be just the kind of fellow you need to keep you alive.

Some patients go on the long trek of finding the perfect doctor because they have lost confidence in the truthfulness of their physician. "Unless I can believe that he's absolutely honest with me, I'll keep looking until I find one who is," said one patient.

Richard C. Cabot, M.D., wrote many years ago: "Truthfulness in diagnosis, I believe, is wholly for the patient's benefit. Most enlightened physicians I know do not cram down the patient's throat all the facts about his case. But when he asks direct questions he is told the truth—no doctor wants to be thought a liar."

Nevertheless, he went on to say: "But a large proportion of honorable physicians and high-minded men DO believe in occasional benevolent deception of their patients. In other words, sometimes they feel it is necessary for the patient's good to be a White Liar or Benevolent Liar."

My own experience has taught me that we can't make generalizations. What is good advice for one patient would be tactless and poor management for the other.

Two Cancer Patients

For example, I recall two patients who had a lump in the breast as the presenting complaint. They went to the same surgeon who had a deserved reputation for being one of the best in the community.

He told one of the women in answer to a direct question: "Yes, I think it's cancer. We won't know definitely until frozen sections are examined at operation. Chances are that your breast will have to be removed." This patient accepted the diagnosis and had a normal recovery.

The other patient's lump was not definitely cancerous in nature. To this patient's direct question the surgeon replied: "I have a hunch that your condition is a benign one. I don't think you will lose your breast. Of course, this is only a guess until the pathologist's report comes back."

In her case, too, breast removal was a necessity because of a positive report of malignancy. Although warned that there was a remote possibility of cancer, she had seemed to wash it out of her mind. She was gay and frolicsome before operation.

A few days afterwards, realizing that her breast had been removed, she went into a deep depression. Later she committed suicide.

After such horrible events, doctors face up to themselves squarely and ask: "Might I have prevented such a tragedy?" An answer is not always forthcoming. What works for one patient is like poison for the next.

Generally, the accepted procedure is to tell the patient the truth. There are exceptions to this rule. Nevertheless, if we hope to have the complete confidence of our patients they must believe that we give them a complete accounting of their illness.

A member of the patient's family will often call up and say: "I understand that John is coming in for a physical checkup. I think you ought to know he is very nervous and concerned about himself. Don't frighten him, doctor. If he has anything wrong, don't tell him. Tell me."

Patient Should Know the Truth

When such a patient comes in, having found that he has heart trouble, I never fail to give him the facts. Often, the wife who phoned will turn back after they have left the inner office, to get the "lowdown" on her husband's condition.

My practice is to invite the husband right back in. In his presence I repeat the diagnosis. I do not believe in "behind-the-back" whispered conversations that keep the patient out of it and raise doubts in his mind about what "really is the matter." This is one way of keeping the patient's confidence in his doctor—which is so necessary for good treatment and unqualified cooperation.

Yes, I believe that patients should be told—but **how** they are told is what matters. There is no need in scaring people unnecessarily.

For example, when a man has had a coronary thrombosis and is anxious for an explanation, I think it is good policy to tell him the truth. "A coronary artery has become blocked off. However, every day your other heart arteries are learning how to take over the added load.

Collateral circulation is the answer to many more years of life."

I have often heard the "truth" put another way: "One of your two main arteries in the heart has been plugged up. You've seen what happens with a rusty pipe. That's what's happened to one of your coronaries."

When the patient asks: "What happens when the other closes up?" the response is sometimes a shrug of the shoulder that indicates "finis" to the worried patient.

You see, I believe that the patient is better off to know the truth, provided his physician takes the time and effort to present it tactfully.

So don't go running off and calling your doctor an alarmist unless he deserves this description. In fact, be thankful if your doctor is candid and frank.

Courageous Patient

I recall one of the finest examples of courage ever exhibited by a patient. It shows how some patients react to frankness and honesty. The story was told to members of the American College of Physicians many years ago during our annual meeting held at Philadelphia. The speaker, Dr. Evarts A. Graham, was one of the foremost chest surgeons of that era.

He said that one day he examined a man who had some chest trouble. Further investigation by x-rays and other methods revealed the cause. The patient had an extensive tumor in one lung. He was traveling a one-way street to extinction. The only thing that might save his life would be complete removal of that lung.

But here was the hitch. It had never been done before.

No surgeon had ever removed an entire lung from a human being. The doctor and his patient had a little talk. In effect, the surgeon said: "You have a dangerous tumor. You will die without operation. You may die *with* operation. But I think you have a chance. I believe you are operable. In all fairness, though, you should know that I've never performed such an extensive operation on a human being. You will be the first—and I hope' not the last. What do you say?"

Without hesitation the man said, "Go ahead. I have complete confidence in you. I know that everything will turn out all right."

You can imagine how this unhesitating decision sustained the spirits of the surgeon. Optimism and manifestations of complete confidence are contagious.

But words are sometimes said in bravado. Perhaps the patient would go home that night and brood. Then he would call up the next morning and say he had changed his mind. It was too dangerous.

However, here is what actually happened as Dr. Graham related it. The patient called the next day to ask if it would be all right if he postponed coming to the hospital for a few days. There were some matters he needed to clean up.

Came the day of the operation, and the surgeon visited with his patient before he was wheeled into the operating room. It was then that he received the necessary jolt of optimism that he needed for the trying task ahead.

Said Dr. Graham, "When you asked for a few days' postponement I thought you were getting cold feet."

The patient sat up in bed and said, "Who me? Not on your life! I suppose I should have told you why I wanted those few extra days before coming into the hospital. You see, I've been having trouble with my dentures lately. So I took time off to have some new ones made. I wanted to have my teeth all taken care of so I wouldn't have to bother about them after the operation."

That's the story of how one patient's optimism spread to his doctor and gave him the courage to remove the first lung in surgical history. I shall never forget this inspiring anecdote on faith and courage.

Footnote: The operation was successful and the patient lived and worked for many years. And the surgeon? Some years later, Dr. Evarts A. Graham died. Ironically, the cause of death was cancer of the lung.

Doctors Are Cheer Leaders

The doctor is often only a cheer leader; it is the patient who "plays the game and gets the bumps." The medical man diagnoses and treats you, but have you ever considered how often he leads you by the hand?

Some of you are as helpless as the elderly lady the little boy scout guides across a crowded street. Others of you are brash and too courageous for your own good. Then it is the doctor's problem to take you in hand, sit you down and read the law to you.

For example, consider this businessman of 44. The diagnosis was easy. He was, as he put it, "just too fat for my own good." He was short and weighed about 220. That was all I could find wrong except a blood pressure that was beginning to climb. In the course of the questioning I asked him if he had any hobbies.

"I have two," he said. "The first is eating. I love to eat. I guess you don't have to be a doctor to recognize that.

My other hobby is playing with children—especially with my own two boys and a girl."

Then it was that I told him how the first hobby would surely destroy the second and more important one. "If you continue to overeat, according to all statistics, you won't live long enough to see your children married. Obesity is slow poison. In the end it will get your heart— or kill you off in one of a half dozen other ways."

He was fashioned of stern stuff. Within four months he lost 40 pounds. At 180 pounds he was a happy man. "Take my word for it," he said, "I'll be down to 150 pounds within 6 months." And he was.

This man was unusual because most obese patients do not react to advice like he did. They need to be cajoled, begged and warned before they will lose. Even so, many of them gain instead of lose. They come back month after month with excuses. "I gained because I had to attend two bachelor dinners and a wedding last week. I'll do better next time."

Patient Needs Moral Support

So the doctor calls a new signal, hoping they will score the next time. He doubles as quarterback and cheer leader. He tells the patient what to do and how to do it. Then he rushes to the sidelines to cheer his patient on. The doctor needs to be patient and humane, otherwise the sick one's last support is gone. The patient leans on his doctor for moral courage more than he realizes.

Many patients have to be saved from themselves. There are two ways to practice medicine. One doctor makes the diagnosis, prescribes and that's that. Whether or not you take the medicine is your own business.

The second doctor not only prescribes, but goes all out to see that you follow his directions. That's the kind of physician to have. Hold on tight; don't let him go, if you're fortunate enough to have him.

Yet, as I have indicated, so many will leave such fine medical men simply because they are impatient. They want immediate action. If they don't get it, they jump on the medical merry-go-round. Soon they have no "one" medical friend they can turn to when problems arise.

Have Good Reasons for Changing Doctors

Make this a rule: don't go from one doctor to another unless you have a good reason. If you are in doubt about the course of your illness and the treatment you are receiving, ask for a consultation, but don't leave him. If you think his fees are getting too high, talk it over. He will make adjustments, I'm sure. But don't leave him. If he keeps you waiting too long for your appointment, talk it out with him, but don't leave him (unless he still keeps you waiting for hours). If he seems abrupt and doesn't take as much time with you as when you first became his patient, complain to him. If he still cuts you short, *leave* him, because an unhurried visit with your doctor is one of the essentials of success. If he doesn't make night calls any more, talk it over. If he can't arrange for suitable coverage, leave him. If he doesn't make any house calls any more, talk it over. If unsatisfactory arrangements are made, leave him.

I hope you understand what I have been trying obliquely to say. There's no contract between you and your doctor for life. He doesn't own you; neither do you own him. You have the right to go from doctor to doctor if the quality of your medical service is much less than it used to be. But I do want to stress this: in the long run he gets the best medical care who has the patience to stick to his doctor—if he is a good one. It's better to be an old patient than a new "case."

Chapter Summary

1. Patients with anxiety about their disease—or imagined disease—often go from doctor to doctor.
2. Many people think a specialist is a doctor who lives "out of town."
3. Diagnostic clinics are of value when treatment or diagnosis at home is questionable or unsatisfactory.
4. Don't jump on the medical merry-go-round.
5. Procrastination may be a threat to life.
6. The ulcer patient often goes looking for trouble unnecessarily because of impatience.
7. It is better to have an "alarmist" who is thorough than a physician who is a poor diagnostician.
8. Patients deserve to know the truth.
9. Review the reactions of the two cancer patients to their operations.
10. Tactfulness should go hand in hand with truthfulness.
11. Reread the unusual story of the courageous patient and the lung operation.

12. The good doctor is like a cheer leader who bolsters the faith of his patient.

13. Many patients need to be saved from themselves.

14. Make sure you have good reason before changing doctors.

The NINTH Commandment: Thou Shalt No Have Too Many Doctors

Forget it IF:

1. You and your family doctor have had a happy relationship for years.
2. You are not an impatient patient.
3. You realize there are no medical geniuses who can quickly control chronic, discomforting illness.
4. You know that complete faith in one doctor is the ideal arrangement between patient and physician.
5. You know that flitting from one doctor to another is not only expensive, but may be life-endangering.

———

NOTE:

Although there is no written contract which legalizes the terms "my doctor" and

Remember it IF:

1. You have been riding th medical merry-go-round
2. You are impatient wit treatment.
3. You have become in censed at your doctor be cause:
   a. His fees are high.
   b. He will not make house calls.
   c. He will not make nigh calls.
   d. He keeps you waiting for hours after you appointment.
   e. He is tactless.
   f. He is an alarmist.
   g. He has violated your confidences.
4. You prefer to shop around until you find a doctor who will give you "good news" instead of "bad."
   a. Even though you need an operation you will

The NINTH Commandment: Thou Shalt Not Have Too Many Doctors (Continued)

"my patient"—this sense of ownership, or close association, is the ideal one where health and life are involved.

Remember it IF:

    seek a doctor who will say you don't.

b. A doctor who will say you don't have to stay in bed for weeks— even though you have coronary thrombosis.

c. A doctor who will say expensive x-rays are unnecessary — even though a suspicious gastric ulcer requires careful observation.

d. Until you find an actual "quack" who will give you promises for cure which an ethical medical man refuses to do.

NOTE:

When in doubt about your doctor's success and methods of treating you, the preferable thing to do is ask for consultation.

10

Thou shalt not

Retire From Your Job

Too Early?

Life can be fun even if you retire at forty-five.

Retirement studies at Cornell University have showed that those who retired voluntarily felt better and lived longer than those who were forced into retirement. My experience in practice bears this out. I recall many examples of people who retired early and reaped the benefits of enjoying life before they got so old their bones were too frail to carry them around.

Consider, for instance, Mr. G., an executive in an industrial firm. I had been taking care of him and his family for about ten years. One day he came in for his yearly physical checkup. I found that except for a mild degree of arthritis in one knee, he was in excellent physical condition for a man of 48.

Wants to Retire Early

"That makes me feel especially good, today," he said. "Have you got time for a little chat and some advice? I've had something on my mind for the past year that I want to talk over. It may seem ridiculous to you, but I was never more serious." Then he looked at me closely to see how I would react and said, "I'm thinking of resigning from my job. I'd like to retire this year."

He seemed grateful that I did not laugh in his face and that I listened to his decision in the same spirit in which it was given.

"What makes you think I would consider it ridiculous?" I asked.

"It's because I know how friends of mine will react and how the community will begin to wonder what's wrong with me. I'm sure most people will think that I've either been kicked out, or that I have heart trouble or something like that. Anybody who even thinks of retiring voluntarily before 65 these days is considered a fool."

"Do *you* consider it a stupid decision?" I asked.

"Of course not," he said. "All I want is your backing and I'll go through with it. My wife is already on my side. My boy and girl are married and settled down, so I have no problems there."

"Before I give you my final word on the matter," I said, "I'd like you to tell me why you want to retire now. Be honest and frank. Unless you have good motivation, your retirement is liable to turn into a fiasco."

"It's simply that I'm fed up with working," he said. "Do I need any other reason?"

"Yes, you do. But I happen to know you have all the qualifications and requirements for early retirement. That's why I go along with you. As far as I'm concerned you can wind up your affairs as quickly as you can, and quit."

The Essential Requirements

Let me explain why I came to that decision. Mr. G. was healthy. My examination had just disclosed that he was in exceptionally good condition for a man his age. I also knew that an inheritance, a large salary over the years, and a wise investment program had made him a wealthy man. There was no question that he and his wife could live comfortably on their income. But perhaps most important of all, our man was fortunate in being a fine, all-around human being.

He was a book-lover and philosopher of sorts. A former athlete in college, the sports page intrigued him as much as did the editorial page. An accomplished pianist, he had a deep love for music. But last, and not least, through study over the years he had become recognized as one of the well-known authorities on modern art. He was an excellent speaker and in great demand to deliver lectures.

What did it all add up to? He had prepared himself physically, economically, and psychologically for retirement. Someone has said that "boredom tires women but kills men." There was no danger that Mr. G. would ever die of boredom.

Mollie Hart in her book *When Your Husband Retires* says: "If a man has any choice in the matter, and if he has a desire to retire or is likely to be required to do so, he should retire voluntarily, not wait until he is forced to, and he should do it before he reaches sixty-five, the age when retirement is customary or mandatory."

Sixty-five? That was too far out in space for Mr. G. even to consider. With my blessings he took the plunge. Note that I didn't say "fateful." Fifteen years later I met my former patient at a dinner party out of town. His grin was wide, his handshake strong, his health apparently excellent. If ever a man deserved the greeting: "You haven't changed a bit"—here was the man. Both he and his wife were the best examples I have ever seen of successful early retirement.

"My wife and I will never forget you for being instrumental in giving us 15 of the happiest years of our life," he said.

He didn't realize—or perhaps he did—that the decision must lie within the individual himself.

Procrastination Was His Enemy

I recall another successful business man who wanted very much to retire when he consulted me at age 50. He was a widower, his six children were married, he lived alone in a large apartment. Although able to afford it, he kept putting off his urge to travel throughout the United States and over the world. He was intensely interested in archaeology. "Someday," he said, "I want to go places and see things."

Came 55, and 60. At each visit he would excuse himself by saying, "I suppose you think I have been talking through my hat all these years. But the truth is that I've been too cowardly to retire when I wanted to. I've always been sensitive to public opinion. My kids have all been after me to get some fun out of life, but I've always wondered what my friends would say if I turned in the office keys before I got to be 65. But now I've really made up my mind. Now that I'm 60 I'm not going to wait any longer."

He died two days later while on his way to a travel agency to make arrangements for a trip. It is difficult to believe, but he had never been outside of a 200-mile radius of the city he lived in all his life.

How Is Your Arithmetic?

The trouble with many of us is that we live as if we were going to be around for another thousand years. Our philosophy seems to be that we will have all the time we want to do the things we want. In addition we are poor mathematicians. Especially in the art of subtraction.

How many at the age of 60, for example, sit down with pencil and paper and subtract that figure from the biblical 70? Few. I guess it's because people do everything possible not to face the reality that some day we will not be here.

But face it. Sixty from 70 leaves 10 years. Suppose you are fortunate and live to be 70 in good health? You do not wheeze with asthma, your joints are not arthritic, your heart does its work so you do not tire on the least exertion.

Have you any plans for those 10 years? What will you do to round out your life: to successfully cap the strains of school and examinations, the pressures of a lifetime of work? As I indicated earlier, the answer must be an individual one. Each has his own mathematical problem, and each may have the correct answer for himself, though it is not a universally applicable answer.

Human beings should be taught to begin their subtraction exercises when in their teens to make plans for retirement. Take 15 from 65 and that leaves a half century of work. The time to make money for retirement, to develop hobbies, and to maintain a healthy body, is when you are young.

Having considered this all-important problem for years, you and you and you will know what it is you want. If your genes are so constituted and arranged that you will be happier if you work until 65, with only five years (or more) for retirement, then I will not be the one to say you are wrong. Many people find in their work their greatest fulfillment. Retirement would only be a ball-and-chain to perpetual boredom.

Against Compulsory Retirement

It is for this reason that I am not in agreement with the antiquated system that prevails in most establishments that compulsory retirement must be the rule when a stipulated age is reached. It grieves and appalls me when I consider the wealth of brains and experience that are squandered every year just because the calendar says a man is through, because his hair is grey, even though his brain is still youthful and resilient.

See, therefore, that I try to be open-minded where the problem of retirement raises its head. But I ask you to try to be likewise. Don't make the mistake of falling into the well-traveled rut. Too many people travel it. They

238 YOUR LIFE TO ENJOY

have got it into their heads that people shouldn't retire too soon. What people? And what is too soon?

Remember the simple arithmetic. It's your life and mine. And the choice is rightfully yours and mine. If your pencil and paper says that 50 years of work is enough for one lifetime and that it deserves 20 years of relaxation, of doing the things you have always wanted to do, then I give you an A on your report card.

If, however, your homework concludes that 65 years of work is the correct formula and your subtraction doesn't upset you when you realize that leaves only five years (more or, often, less) for retirement, then I will mark you an A, too.

If your calculations indicate you will be happier with 30 years of retirement, I will even more readily give you an A—not only for effort—but for good sense.

Favors Early Retirement

I suppose you have guessed that I am in favor of earlier retirement than the universally accepted deadline ot 62 or 65. To me these are false demarcation lines. Most people, if pressed for an honest answer, will tell you they'd like to retire much earlier than in the middle sixties.

"Of course," says Mr. K., "who, in his right mind, will admit that he enjoys being thrown out of bed every morning by the clang of the alarm? Who likes to be tied down every day by a growing list of appointments with all kinds of people—those you like, despise, or think stupid? Who but a moron will say that he likes to rush through breakfast to catch the train into the city or the bus to the office?

"You are willing to put up with it when you are raising

a family, paying off the mortgage on the house, and trying to make a place for yourself in the community. But isn't it human to get a little tired of all this rigmarole when you have been at it for so many years?

"As for me, if I could afford it, I'd quit tomorrow. I'm 45 and I've worked hard all my life since kindergarten. I don't think it's too early to retire at my age. But my tough luck is that I'll probably have to stay in harness until they put me out to pasture."

No Secret for Longevity

Ask a dozen or more people who have lived to the age of 100 the secret of their longevity. How did you manage to get there? What did or didn't you do to reach the three-figure mark?

Good heredity? One says: "My mother and father died before 50. There is no history of longevity in my family."

Another: "I have smoked since I can remember."

Another: "I have been at least 40 pounds overweight since my teens."

Another: "There wasn't a day that I didn't take more than a nip of whiskey."

Another: "Whenever I felt worry coming on I stopped it by going to sleep."

Another: "Exercise? I've been lazy all my life. I wouldn't take an extra step unless I had to."

Another: "Special diet? Not for me. I figured anything I liked was all right to eat. Fats, fried foods, coffee. I ate and drank what I liked. Examinations? I haven't been to a doctor in fifty years."

On his 101st birthday, during a recent interview in

Connecticut, the spirited "youngster" gave these reasons for his attainment of old age: "Be a Democrat, smoke and don't diet."

Of course, there were those who never drank or smoked, who had their special diets, who went to the doctor regularly, who kept their weight within normal limits, who exercised to keep fit.

But you will note that there is no blanket formula which is good enough to cover each and every one of us. Thereby hangs a tale. Medicine may not yet really have the answer to the question of what is best for YOU and ME.

Individual Problem

This is surely true where proper time for retirement is the problem. *You* must furnish the answer. Resolve to quit before you are physically or mentally worn out. I know you will be faced with many fears and uncertainties. These, more than anything else, prevent so many from retiring at the time they most want to.

For example, here are some of the fears that people encounter who are considering retirement, or at least "dreaming" about it.

After a while will I find myself sitting, just sitting, and twiddling my thumbs?

Will the business go to pot? Am I expendable?

Will I miss the daily challenge?

Just what does retirement accomplish?

What will people think? How about the loss of prestige in the smaller groups and in the community?

How tough will it be for me and my wife to make the

transition from full days to empty days, from old friends to new?

All these doubts and anxieties are the natural questions that arise in the mind of any person who is making a drastic change in his way of life. They are to be expected. If you are going forward in your car you must stop before you go into reverse. No abrupt change is entirely smooth.

Some Good Reasons

Nevertheless, the change of direction is often absolutely necessary if your life is to be fulfilled. For example, if you work in daily tension you should consider retirement if you are in your fifties or sixties. If your business or profession is such that it is a welter of frustrations and unhappy irritations, consider retirement. Also if you have been in the grip of fatigue day after day for months, retirement may be the answer. If you want to live out the rest of your existence in reasonable happiness, you must make the break. Like anything else, it seems absolutely impossible to undertake until you actually try it.

Many people don't go through with retirement because they are guilt-stricken. Leave my business in the lurch? Give up on community affairs? Leave my friends? Such are the ones who do not realize that each and every one of us is expendable. Too much self-importance is a common cause for lopsided guilt-feelings.

Doctor Retires Early

A number of years ago I read a magazine article by a prominent obstetrician who was retiring at the age of 55.

He was looking forward to hearing telephones ring without having to answer, to turning calendar pages without wondering if a baby would be on time, to going to sleep without the inevitable interruptions at night, to tending his garden.

As I recall it he said something like this: "What I can't understand is the feeling of hostility and underlying animosity that I detect in a number of my old patients whom I served so conscientiously for many years. Some have come right out with it, while others just think it: Aren't you letting us down by retiring now?

"I didn't even answer them. If they couldn't understand that a doctor isn't all machine, that he is at least part human being with needs and wishes and dreams of his own, then it's just too bad. I was in practice over 30 years, during which time I gave of myself as much as a human being can. I delivered thousands of babies. I operated. I consoled. I gave physical and mental comfort. My conscience is clear, even if I never open another medical book again or never see another patient. I've seen too many old, feeble and sick doctors with their little black bags frantically trying to hold on to their practices while the world and life passes them by. That's not for me. Call me selfish if you will—but I think the Man Upstairs will rule you out of order."

It Is Later Than You Think

Many years ago, Dr. Frederick Loomis wrote in his book *The Bond Between Us,* "Enjoy yourself, it is later than you think." This is the most quoted line. But he also wrote:

Many years have been added to the average expectation of life, but each individual's fate is still a hazard. The most valuable people around us have lived largely for others. This seems the time to remind them that they will have more years, and happier ones, to do good for others, if they start right now to do something for themselves, to go places and to do things which they have looked forward to for years, to give those who love them the happiness of seeing them enjoy some of the rewards which they have earned, to replace competition with a bit of contemplation.

Not in a vacation, short or prolonged, but only in retirement can you hope to gain such benefits.

Dare to live! Often the supreme dare is to retire early. It is preferable to be called the black sheep than to conform to a deadly routine because the flock follows it blindly.

Your time for retirement may be now, later, or never. However, if it is *now* and you do not take advantage of the gift of the Gods, you may never have this opportunity again.

The saddest words in the language—any language—are: "If I had only . . . !"

It's not the things we *did* but the things we *didn't* do that give us the greatest remorse.

Chapter Summary

1. Those who retire voluntarily feel better and live longer than those who are forced into it.
2. Reread the case history of the patient who retired at 48.
3. There are three essential preparatory measures for

successful retirement: the economical, physical and psychological.

4. "Boredom tires women but kills men."

5. Reread the sad case of the man whose enemy was procrastination.

6. The need for retirement often can be brought into clear focus by simple subtraction.

7. The time to prepare for retirement is in the teens.

8. Compulsory retirement of able individuals is both cruel and a senseless waste of precious brain-power and experience.

9. Only YOU can correctly answer if you will be happier with 5 years of retirement or with 20.

10. There is no blanket rule for attaining the age of 100; neither is there one all-encompassing rule on the proper age for retirement.

11. Don't be influenced against retiring by what others may think. It is a peculiarly personal problem. If you have good reasons, go ahead and *dare to live*.

12. "It is later than you think" is an evident truth, apparently not believed by the majority.

The TENTH Commandment: Thou Shalt Not Retire Too Early

Forget it IF:

1. You have already retired.
2. You are physically, economically and psychologically able.
3. You have worked hard and have made a gratifying work-contribution to the world you live in.
4. You are retiring to something. You have developed one or more absorbing hobbies.
5. Your wife is willing to take the plunge.
6. Work is no longer fun. You are under daily stress and have become irritable and chronically tired.
7. You have the courage to do what is best for you and yours in spite of unsympathetic attitude of friends and community.

Remember it IF:

1. All you have known is work.
2. You have no outside interests or hobbies.
3. Your wife doesn't want you to retire. An unhappy wife is more than a drop of vinegar in the honey jar of retirement.
4. You haven't enough money.
5. You are too sick to enjoy the fun and excitement of active retirement.
6. You are filled with anxiety about changing your comfortable, "old shoe" way of life and substituting many new and untried factors.
7. You love your job so much that you are certain that retirement would "bore you to death."

The TENTH Commandment: Thou Shalt Not Retire Too Early (Continued)

NOTE:

One's age is not the important factor; but need and preparation for retirement are. Retirement may be a failure at 65 and a success at 45. Those who dare to live get the most out of life. The saddest people I have known are those who say when they reach 60-65: "I wanted to retire years ago but I didn't have the guts."

NOTE:

The man who wants to work until 65 is no fool; but neither is the one who wants to quit at 50. Each of us has his own likes and dislikes; and his own dreams. For some, work is a nightmare, and retirement a heaven-on-earth. For others, vice versa.

Some jump into retirement as carelessly as others do into a shallow pool. Be careful before you make the leap.

Retiring from your job is as important as choosing it in the first place. Each decision requires ability and good sense.

Sudden impulse rarely achieves the goal of happy retirement.

Conclusion

How To Realize Your Happiness Potential

Review and consider carefully the Ten Commandments I have enumerated and discussed. If you can honestly determine how they apply to you—and take immediate, proper action—it is conceivable that, from this very day, you will have immeasurably increased your happiness potential.

If you have read the chapters carefully, reviewed the summations at the end of each, and made the necessary decision to **Forget** a Commandment or **Remember** it, you will have taken more than one giant stride toward fulfillment. For I hope I have convinced you that no life can be a full success without health.

As a parting note from author to reader, I ask you to

read what I say—and resist the temptation to put the book aside and go on living in fear. You have come so far, come a little farther.

For example, consider Chapter I again. (1st Commandment: **Thou Shalt Not Take Cholesterol.**) I hope I have been able to rid you, on the one hand, of "cholesterolophobia"; and on the other, convinced you that common sense dictates a play-it-safe attitude if you are a potential candidate for atherosclerosis. In other words, if there are no contra-indications, for pity's sake sit down to your steak dinner with dessert and all the fixings and enjoy your eating conscience-free. Too many wear the heavy yoke of needless dieting because of the cholesterol scare. Eating an ice cream cone or pouring heavy cream into a cup of coffee should not feel like a headlong journey into perdition and extinction.

Likewise, neither should patients with known high cholesterol readings and a poor family history laugh off its importance in the maintenance of good health. Such people need to remember the Commandment.

In Chapter 2 (2nd Commandment: **Thou Shalt Not Be Lazy**) you will find sufficient reasons for being thankful that the good Lord put some lazy bones in your body. It will take much more convincing than comes out of Washington to throw your skeleton and muscles around in the belief that forty-plus Americans require daily exercise to keep fit and healthy.

Chapter 3 (3rd Commandment: **Thou Shalt Not Take Tobacco**) takes the sting out of your pipe-stem as you light up for an after-dinner smoke. For many tobacco is a poison, for others a threat, and for still others nothing but an unalloyed joy as one of the pleasures of life.

If you reread Chapter 4 (4th Commandment: **Thou**

Shalt Not Have Anxiety) you will accept the fact that no one is free from anxiety; that each one of us lives in the shadow of the bomb. But you will also know that, although worry cannot be neutralized by the wave of a philosophical wand, we can learn to be happy if we recognize stress for what it is and take proper steps to take it by the hand as a friend rather than as an enemy.

Chapter 5 bears rereading a few times (5th Commandment: **Thou Shalt Not Take Alcohol**). For here you may have to weigh carefully my reasons for advising you to take alcohol every day. It requires persuasive powers (which one reading may not furnish) to convince you to take alcohol for your own good when you have been brought up believing that it is an evil and a universal poison. For many the time will come when they agree that a martini or other drink before dinner has changed the course of their lives for the better. And the potential alcoholics will know that I am not blind to alcohol's menace, either.

In Chapter 6 (6th Commandment: **Thou Shalt Not Eat Too Much**)—which you need only skim over—is the restatement of the potential evils of excess weight.

In Chapter 7 (7th Commandment: **Thou Shalt Not Be Under Too Great Stress**) you will rediscover that the mere act of living is stressful. You will realize that it is as unnatural to fight against "natural" stress as it is to fight against taking nourishment or breathing. But you will learn to distinguish between stress you can live with and stress you must abolish.

Chapter 8 (8th Commandment: **Thou Shalt Not Become a Victim of Your Emotions**). If after reading this chapter you still doubt that the emotions exert their effects (good and bad) upon the body, and vice versa, then your name must really be Thomas.

In Chapter 9 (9th Commandment: **Thou Shalt Not Have Too Many Doctors**) you come face to face with the realization that the patient on the medical merry-go-round, seeking frantically for the "perfect" doctor, will find not only disillusionment, but will actually endanger his health and life by this continual search. Of all the Commandments, this is one of the most important: for it embodies the realization that the finest doctor-patient relationship ensues only when the patient shows his trust by being steadfast and not flitting from doctor to doctor. Disease grows strong on indecision and procrastination—and too many doctors can poison the broth rather than just spoil it.

In Chapter 10 (10th Commandment: **Thou Shalt Not Retire From Your Job Too Early**) you will find reason enough to stay put on your job even if you are over 65 (if they let you); or, pack up your belongings and scoot out of the office forever, in your late forties or fifties—convinced that you have prepared for retirement psychologically, physically, emotionally and financially.

Having carefully reread or skimmed the preceding chapters it will begin to dawn upon you that my chief purpose —the underlying theme of the book—is to stress the need to face up to yourself as a human being in relation to yourself and your environment, to be aware that the Biblical age of 70 (ten years, give or take) is our viable limit in this worldly sphere, that life is a one-way street, that we live only once.

All this being evident and true beyond a doubt, it follows as the night the day, that nothing is more important than to *stop being scared* and remember it's YOUR LIFE TO ENJOY.

The celebrated natural approach to health, beauty, dieting and vitality...

HERBS, HEALTH & COOKERY

Claire Loewenfeld and Philippa Back

"A valuable guide to the uses of herbs, medicinal as well as culinary. The large cookbook section provides more than 300 easy-to-follow recipes that bring the most exotic as well as the most subtle flavorings within the reach of every cook."

—*News American* (Baltimore)

"Introduces herbs to the novice, giving uses and health-giving properties; their role in food preparations and medicinal teas; and their use in the care of skin, hair and eyes. In these times of synthetic flavors of over-processed foods, it is refreshing to use savory herbs to whet the appetite." —*Natural Food and Farming*
A575–95¢

THE INCREDIBLE KRUPPS

Norbert Muhlen

The fascinating story of the gigantic munitions empire that stormed through history. A stunning portrait of the intimate scandals and bizarre perversions that were essential parts of the Krupp family. A550–95¢

A detailed city-by-city guide to hundreds of places selling good original art for as low as $10!

BUYING ART ON A BUDGET
Joanna Eagle

Learn what to buy: Develop your own individualistic taste in prints, drawings, watercolors, modern and contemporary paintings, antiques, primitive and Oriental craft and sculpture.

Discover where to buy: Detailed information on galleries, museums, auctions, universities, department stores, mail-order outlets, installment-buying places and many other sources.

Find out what to do after making the purchase: How to frame and display your pieces, how to care for them, how to make them an important part of your home and life.

"An excellent book on art collecting."
— *Publishers' Weekly*
A574—$1.25

———————

THE POWER OF FAITH HEALING
Shaw Desmond

Revealed—the secrets of the great healers and their magical cures. You could be a natural-born faith healer unknown to yourself. Find out in this amazing book. A533—75¢

A panoramic guide to forbidden erotic works...

THE ENCYCLOPEDIA OF EROTICA

Edited by Dr. Paul J. Gillette

Artworks whose primary focus is on sexual desire, activity or behavior, selected by the editor as significant examples of erotic literature, comprise the selection of erotica in this collection.

Ranging from classics to best-selling novels of today, this fantastic volume contains, in their entirety, long-suppressed works like Ovid's *Art of Love*, Mark Twain's *1601*, de Maupassant's *Forbidden Fruit*, as well as lengthy excerpts from well-known books (*The Memoirs of Dolly Morton*, *Grushenka*, *City of Night*, *Candy*) and underground classics (*White Thighs*, *The Whipping Club*, *The Virgin of Orleans*, *The Amours of a Musical Student*). A497--$1.50